AIDS and the Social Sciences

AIDS and the Social Sciences

Common Threads

Richard Ulack and William F. Skinner
Editors

THE UNIVERSITY PRESS OF KENTUCKY

Copyright © 1991 by The University Press of Kentucky

Scholarly publisher for the Commonwealth,
serving Bellarmine College, Berea College, Centre
College of Kentucky, Eastern Kentucky University,
The Filson Club, Georgetown College, Kentucky
Historical Society, Kentucky State University,
Morehead State University, Murray State University,
Northern Kentucky University, Transylvania University,
University of Kentucky, University of Louisville,
and Western Kentucky University.

Editorial and Sales Offices: Lexington, Kentucky 40508-4008

Library of Congress Cataloging-in-Publication Data

AIDS and the social sciences : common threads / edited by Richard
  Ulack and William F. Skinner.
        p.   cm.
    Proceedings of a symposium held in October 1989 on the University
  of Kentucky campus.
    ISBN 0-8131-1760-7
    1. AIDS (Disease)—Social aspects—Congresses.   I. Ulack,
  Richard, 1942-   II. Skinner, William Francis.
    RA644.A25A354   1991
  362.1'969792—dc20   91-13348

This book is printed on acid-free paper meeting
the requirements of the American National Standard
for Permanence of Paper for Printed Library Materials. ♾

Contents

vi   Contents

Tables & Figures

Tables

Figures

Preface

In the spring of 1989 we asked our colleague Gary Shannon, a noted medical georapher who is currently conducting research on AIDS (Shannon and Pyle 1989; Shannon, Pyle, and Bashur 1990), if he would be interested in helping organize a seminar or symposium on AIDS. The College of Arts and Sciences at the University of Kentucky had issued a call for proposals for funding through its Enrichment Fund and it was in response that we developed the proposal. We proposed that a two-day symposium be held on the University of Kentucky campus in October 1989. The symposium was to be titled "AIDS and the Social Sciences: A Public Symposium on Research Agendas and Applications" and was to include several workshop sessions and a series of about eight major speakers who were noted experts from the social sciences and related applied fields. The symposium, we were later to discover, was unique in that it was one of the very first that specifically addressed AIDS and the social sciences and included participants from most relevant fields of inquiry. The major speakers came from geography, sociology, anthropology, psychology, and social work and represented academe, federal government agencies, and local agencies. Workshop organizers and participants likewise included representatives of these same disciplinary and institutional backgrounds and also included persons living with AIDS.

The College of Arts and Sciences Enrichment Fund awarded us $4,000 under the condition that we find matching funds. Within a week or so, more than sufficient matching funds were committed by a variety of other units, both on campus and off. In addition to the College of Arts and Sciences, cosponsors of the symposium were the University of Kentucky's Department of Geography, Department of Sociology, Department of Behavioral

Science (College of Medicine), Department of Anthropology, Department of Psychology, Department of Political Science, Center for Prevention Research, Martin School of Public Administration, Office of the Vice Chancellor for Research and Graduate Studies, and Graduate School. Other organizations donating funds and other forms of support were the Lexington-Fayette County Health Department, the AIDS Crisis Task Force of Lexington (ACT-Lexington), the Fayette County HIV/AIDS Program, and the East Central AIDS Education and Training Center (ECAETC).

Several other individuals donated considerable time and effort and became an integral part of the symposium core planning group. These were Dr. Phyllis Nash of the Department of Behavioral Science; Judy Stephenson of ECAETC; Sandy Joseph, AIDS manager, Fayette County HIV/AIDS Program; and Marcy Rosenbaum, graduate student in the Department of Anthropology.

A portion of the AIDS Memorial Quilt, a gigantic quilt with panels memorializing individual AIDS deaths, was on public display throughout the symposium. We would like to express our gratitude and thanks to Tom Tollman and his friend from the Dayton, Ohio, chapter of the NAMES Project (a non-profit foundation whose primary activity involves the display and care of the quilt) for their efforts in making this possible. This was the first public display of a portion of the quilt in Kentucky. The display helped to create an interest in beginning a NAMES chapter in this state.

Many other individuals, of course, helped in a variety of ways in putting together the symposium, and to all we say thanks. These included workshop participants Dr. Ivan Banks, Kentucky State University; Beverly Henderson, Women's Center of Central Kentucky; Ron Jerrell, president of the Kentucky-Indiana People with AIDS Coalition (KIPWAC) and secretary-treasurer of the National Association of People with AIDS (NAPWA); Donna C. Vaughn, Hemophilia Program, Kentucky Commission for Handicapped Children; Keith Cecil, University of Kentucky Medical Center; Eric Clifton, person living with AIDS; geography graduate students Roger Miller, Karen Falconer, Gerry Thomas, and Adrian Smith; and sociology graduate student Shireen Rajaram. Finally, we would like to thank Joseph-Beth Booksellers for its excellent display of books on AIDS and staff assistants Joyce Rieman and Betty Jo Friskney of the Department of Geography and Melissa Forsyth of the Department of Sociology.

This book is dedicated to Kentuckians who have died of AIDS, to their families and friends, and to those living with AIDS.

1

Introduction

RICHARD ULACK

The literature on Acquired Immunodeficiency Syndrome (AIDS) is voluminous and growing, as the lengthy bibliography at the end of this volume attests. That this is so is not at all surprising given the tremendous importance of the topic and the impact that it has had, and will continue to have for the foreseeable future, on the world's population. Since its discovery in the United States in the early 1980s, over 160,000 AIDS cases have been reported in this country (through December 1990), and an estimated 1.5 million people in the United States are infected with the virus believed to be responsible: Human Immunodeficiency Virus Type 1, or more simply HIV-1. Cases of AIDS-related deaths worldwide reported to the World Health Organization number over 150,000, and the number of HIV-1-infected persons is conservatively placed at between 5 and 10 million.

Prior to October 1985 and the AIDS-related death of movie star Rock Hudson, few had paid attention to the disease even though some 12,000 Americans were already dead or dying of AIDS (Shilts 1988, xxi–xxiii). This lack of concern largely resulted from the fact that AIDS was perceived as a disease that afflicted homosexuals, a population that most politicians, government workers, and health officials tended to avoid. A few medical doctors and health officials, however, recognized that there was a potential tragedy in the making in the early 1980s. Randy Shilts in his *And the Band Played On* recognizes these early "dramatis personae"; indeed, one of them, Bill Darrow, is an author in this volume (Shilts 1988, xiii). But after 1985, AIDS was recognized as the epidemic that it was and as a national (indeed, global) tragedy. In 1985, 10,875 cases of AIDS were reported to the Centers for Disease Control (CDC), and in 1989, the number reported had increased to over 29,000, or by 168 percent. Of the more than 128,000 AIDS cases reported through March 1990, 90.1 percent were male; in terms of race, 53.1 percent were non-Hispanic whites, 27.6 percent were non-Hispanic blacks, and 15.6 percent were Hispanic; in terms of age, 80.1 percent were between the ages of 20 and 44, and 1.7 percent (2,192) were under 13 years of age (Centers for Disease Control 1990a).

In addition to the gay population, other groups soon began to be identified as having AIDS (table 1.1). The largest of these groups is intravenous (IV) drug users; however, hemophiliacs and others, including women and children who contracted the virus through blood transfusions, are groups whose numbers are rapidly increasing. Belinda Mason, a Kentuckian and member of the National Commission on AIDS who died in 1991, and 12-year-old Ryan White, who died in 1990, are but two of the better-known persons in the latter category.

In addition to being found among all race, sex, and age categories, AIDS is widespread geographically throughout the United States, although clearly the largest metropolitan areas have the largest number of cases (table 1.2). Initially a bicoastal disease limited largely to the metropolitan giants of New York, San Francisco, and Los Angeles, AIDS has since diffused to other cities, smaller towns, and rural areas throughout the nation, as is so aptly presented in the chapter by the geographer Peter Gould. In a recent speech given to the U.S. House of Representatives, Belinda Mason stated, "By 1991, 80 percent of all new AIDS cases will be outside major metropolitan areas. The 1990s will be the decade that AIDS comes home—to the small communities and quiet country towns of the Midwest and South" (*Lexington Herald-Leader,* Feb. 25, 1990, F3.) Clearly, people everywhere need to learn all they can about the AIDS epidemic as it continues to diffuse throughout the country and the world and among all population groups.

Table 1.1. Total Reported AIDS Cases in the U.S. by Exposure Category through March 1990

Exposure category	AIDS cases	
	Number	Percent
Male homosexual/bisexual contact	72,833	57.7
IV drug use (female/heterosexual male)	23,049	18.3
Hemophilia/coagulation disorder	688	0.5
Heterosexual contact	5,936	4.7
Receipt of blood transfusion, blood component, tissue	3,040	2.4
Other/undetermined	4,268	3.4
Single mode of exposure subtotal	(109,814)	(87.0)
Male homosexual/bisexual contact; IV drug use	7,872	6.2
IV drug use; heterosexual contact	2,987	2.4
All other combinations	5,454	4.4
Multiple modes of exposure subtotal	(16,313)	(13.0)
Total	126,127	100.0

Source: Centers for Disease Control 1990a.

The major objective of the symposium, and therefore of this volume, is to inform, educate, and enhance the understanding of the social science community about the etiology, spread, and prevention of AIDS. As initially envisioned, the symposium from which the chapters in this volume are derived had several local goals, including contributing to the education of social scientists and other interested persons regarding the dimensions of the problem and the current status of related research, developing a specified social sciences research strategy, and establishing coordinated and long-term efforts among social scientists at the University of Kentucky and in the Lexington community. By bringing together noted experts from the social science disciplines, relevant government and agency representatives, and persons living with AIDS and their advocates, we felt that new insights into the research needs and perhaps even a substantive multidisciplinary research agenda might be forthcoming. It is still too soon to evaluate how successful we were in this, but the October 1989 symposium generated considerable local interest. The chapters in this volume include all the papers that were presented; in some cases the papers have been updated and expanded.

The chapter by geographer Gary Shannon addresses the important question regarding the various theories about the geographic origin of AIDS (Euro-American, Haitian, and African) and finds "there exists no conclusive scientific evidence for locating the exact origin of the HIV." Rather, Shannon's search for origins reveals that "we are woefully lacking in our understanding of behavior patterns important to the transmission of HIV." This paper (as well as others in this volume) emphasizes the importance of cooperative efforts among social and behavioral scientists if we are to begin to answer the important questions, such as those addressed in this paper.

Peter Gould states that "we have virtually no idea of [the] extent [of AIDS] in geographic space." Following a cogent discussion of the importance of the geographical perspective to an understanding of AIDS, map sequences in his chapter dramatically demonstrate the diffusion of AIDS from the large urban areas to the rural areas of selected states (Ohio and Pennsylvania). Such maps (and especially the map sequences being made for presentation on television) show clearly the geographical dynamics of AIDS and are designed to be used in educational intervention campaigns. Gould questions important data and methodological issues including confidentiality and the inappropriateness of some mathematical approaches.

Ernie Drucker's chapter examines the tremendous impact (an "unparalleled disaster") that AIDS is having on New York City's poor population and its dire implications for the city's large underclass population. Nearly 20 percent of all reported AIDS cases in the United States have been in the New York metropolitan area (table 1.2). Drucker discusses the relationship between family and social support systems and the great need for the further development of public support systems to facilitate early detection, medical treatment, and, ultimately, prevention.

Edwin Hackney's chapter examines the impact of and com-

Table 1.2. Total Reported AIDS Cases in the U.S. by Geographical Region through March 1990

	AIDS cases	
Geographical region	Number	Percent
New York Metropolitan region	24,935	19.4
Los Angeles Metropolitan region	8,739	6.8
San Francisco Metropolitan region	7,894	6.2
All other Metropolitan regions >500,000 population	67,402	52.5
Urban areas <500,000 and rural areas	19,349	15.1
Total	128,319	100.0

Source: Centers for Disease Control 1990a.

munity responses to the epidemic in a much smaller community that so far has been less affected by AIDS—Lexington, Kentucky. The ambivalence, lack of support, and homophobia of most in the community is apparent. There is considerable ignorance about the epidemic in Lexington, no doubt partly because of the low incidence of AIDS in Fayette County (Lexington). As of the end of March 1990, 362 cases of AIDS had been reported for the state of Kentucky, and 43 (12 percent) of those were in Fayette County. Not unlike Drucker in his recommendations for much larger New York City, Hackney strongly urges increased public support and funding, as well as changes in attitude among the public, including the ambivalence that exists among professionals working with AIDS.

Bill Darrow's chapter explores how the principles of sociology and epidemiology can be applied to an understanding of AIDS through the case study approach. He also examines recent studies involving heterosexual transmission of HIV, discusses HIV prevalance among prostitutes, and offers suggestions for future research. Darrow discusses the increasing incidence of the disease in smaller towns and rural areas of the United States, a recurrent theme in a number of the chapters.

Ron Stall outlines the epidemic as it has affected San Francisco, where over 6 percent of all reported AIDS cases in the United States have occurred (table 1.2). Much of Stall's paper is devoted to psychosocial aspects of AIDS research from the perspective of his disciplinary training in anthropology. Stall makes a strong case for inductive theory building, suggesting that "it is required if we are to understand the conditions under which cost-effective and humane care can be given to those who suffer from HIV infection."

The chapter by Doug Feldman evaluates the current AIDS situation in central and East Africa and the way in which African governments and international agencies are responding to the crisis. Clearly, the health and well-being of the entire continent are being challenged by AIDS, and this challenge needs to be responded to quickly.

Beth Schneider's chapter examines AIDS and women and children in the context of "issues, situational contexts, institutional spheres, and policy domains that beg for social scientific and sociological investigation." She develops a strong case for the need for a research agenda for women and children that addresses the unique problems of these groups, such as the oppression and relative powerlessness that women have within existing social and political structures.

In the final chapter, Ernestine Vanderveen takes a "systematic look at trends in the expenditure of fiscal resources by the federal government on AIDS-related activities." She explores how AIDS research and funding patterns have evolved in the Public Health Service, identifies the relative importance of funding by the various federal agencies, and speculates on some of the issues, concerns, and options that will impact future directions and funding. Among the options discussed are the reordering of research priorities and working toward developing a health care system that can handle a major crisis such as AIDS. Whatever option is followed, however, the chapter concludes that a balanced knowledge base can only be developed through "an integrated and equal partnership among the biological, behavioral, and social sciences." This, it seems to us, is a major theme throughout this volume.

Taken together, the nine chapters are good examples of and provide an excellent overview for the research directions and agendas from various social science perspectives. Most call for increased cooperative efforts among the social and behavioral science disciplines since findings can be greatly enhanced only through such research. All the authors offer some answers, but, more importantly, they identify directions for future research and ask vital questions that need to be examined. One of the more important contributions of this volume may be the many questions that are raised, questions best answered through multidisciplinary dialogue.

2

AIDS: A Search for Origins

GARY W. SHANNON

According to Sir Fred Hoyle and his colleague, the Human Immunodeficiency Virus (HIV) is of extraterrestrial origin (McClure and Schulz 1989; Hoyle and Wickramasingke 1990). It has also been suggested that the virus was created either deliberately as a biological warfare weapon by the "doctors of death" at Fort Dietrich, Maryland, or accidentally by molecular biologists in a recombinant research laboratory of some sort in the USSR or Eastern Europe (Executive Intelligence Review 1988). A hypothesis of a similar genre links the HIV to an African strain of swine virus causing deadly fever among Cuban hogs, the source of the virus being either importation of infected stock or the direct and malicious contamination of the Cuban hogs financed by the Central Intelligence Agency (Leibowitch 1985). Others maintain that perhaps it was not venereal syphilis at all but the HIV infection that Columbus's sailors brought back from Hispaniola or Haiti in 1493 (Andre 1987). A "Euro-American" origin has been "traced" based on the similarity of the HIV to a virus (visna-maedi) found in northern European sheep and the implied transfer of the virus to humans by sexual contact between human males and sheep (Kantner and Pankey 1987). These hypotheses—admittedly, some of the more exotic ones that have been posited—illustrate the wide range of proposed origins for the HIV, from outer space to a petri dish, from Columbus to bestiality.

In this chapter I will briefly review three of the more prominent hypotheses and related evidence pertaining to the search for the origins of the HIV, identify difficulties and the potential contribution of social sciences research in this area, and present a general research strategy for comment and discussion.

The Virus and the Search

In the scientific community, though skeptics remain and their dissent is acknowledged here (Duesberg 1987), there is general acceptance of the Human Immunodeficiency Virus (HIV) as the disease agent underlying the Acquired Immunodeficiency Syndrome (AIDS). Since the early stages of the epidemic, and particularly since the recognition of the pandemic of HIV infection, one of the central issues has been the search for the origin of the virus.

Only by conducting a search for its origin and accumulating evidence can the history and geography of the infection be more completely elaborated and demonstrated. And more importantly, the search is vital to understanding the evolution and transmission of the HIV and how to control the biological and social mechanisms of the virus (McClure and Schulz 1989; Essex 1989). The future prevention of AIDS is the real challenge, and understanding the origins of HIV and the mechanisms of its transfer may eventually contribute to its control.

To date, the origin of HIV remains a mystery. As with other diseases, such as venereal syphilis mentioned earlier, the search for the origins of HIV will continue for years and we may never know its actual origin with complete assurance. Nevertheless, it is important to make the effort.

The search is not without its difficulties and complications. Throughout much of history, ethnocentricity, flaming political and social passions and animosity have underlain assigning "blame" for the origins of various diseases, especially those carrying the social stigma generally attached to diseases associated with sexual behavior.

Certainly, in the past a certain level of ethnocentricity was evident in statements describing and attempts to locate the "index location" of a particular disease. In the eighteenth and nineteenth centuries, for example, yellow fever was known as the "Malady of Siam." During the syphilis pandemic in Europe in the late fifteenth and early sixteenth centuries, to the Turks syphilis was the disease of the Christians, to the English it was the French Pox, to the French the Neapolitan disease, to the Italians the Spanish disease, and to the Spanish it was known as the "evil of the island of Hispaniola" brought to Spain by Columbus's crew upon their return from the New World in 1493 (Winslow 1980; Andre 1987). As we shall see, in some early as well as a few recent statements pertaining to the origin of HIV there is evidence that the situation is not much changed. Certain groups of people and nations are "blamed" for somehow "originating" the virus. Frequently, in response, those being "blamed" will marshall "evidence" to either deflect the accusation or lay the blame at the doorstep of others. The process thereby becomes contentious.

Further compounding the problem of searching for the origin of HIV, especially in the early stages of the pandemic, was the lack of cooperation by certain nations and the denial of the existence of HIV-related health problems in some countries. In addition, some early testing procedures on stored sera to detect the presence of antibodies to HIV, the major basis for designating and defining an index region, were later found to be imprecise—providing a rather high percentage of false-positive indications of the presence of HIV antibodies in some cases. This has necessitated the reassessment of earlier statements regarding the distribution of the virus. Finally, the virus itself, as well as associated conditions and diseases, continues to evolve, leading to periodic redefinition of the virus indicator conditions. The clinical expression of infection appears increasingly complex. The types of opportunistic infections and neoplasms may vary not only in populations of different geographic origin but also according to the way the HIV infection was acquired (Piot and Colebunders 1987). Therefore, the distribution of HIV infection indicated by the presence or absence of certain presumed related conditions and diseases changes also.

Despite these obstacles, it is important to assess and attempt to integrate contemporary information pertaining to the geographic origin and diffusion if HIV—acknowledging, of

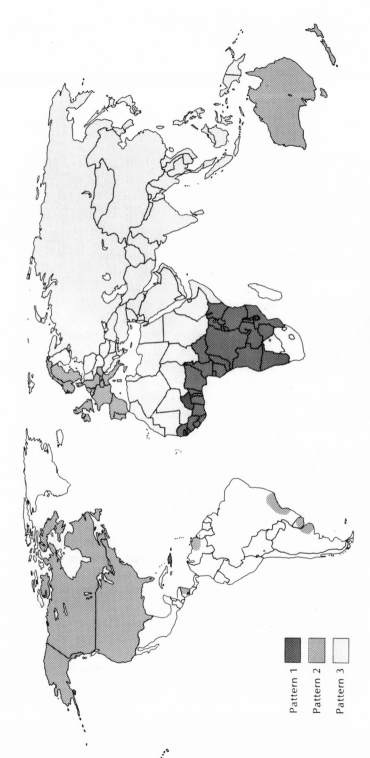

Figure 2.1. Global Patterns of HIV Infection

Pattern 1

Pattern 2

Pattern 3

course, that as our knowledge increases, conclusions regarding the geographic origins may change.

Global Patterns of Infection

Though fewer than ten years have elapsed since identification of the pandemic of HIV infection, on a global scale, three broad but distinct patterns of infection have been distinguished (Von Reyn and Mann 1987; Mann 1988; Torrey, Way, and Rowe 1988). (See figure 2.1).

PATTERN I. The first pattern is found largely in sub-Saharan Africa and increasingly in Latin America, especially the Caribbean. HIV infection likely began to spread extensively during the mid-1970s. However, sexual transmission is predominantly heterosexual and the male to female ratios of infection are approximately 1:1. In this pattern the spread by intravenous drug use is relatively rare, but the virus may be spread by the repeated use of needles without sterilization and the common use of other skin-piercing instruments for medical or ritual purposes. Because of the increased percentage of women infected, perinatal transmission is a major problem in some areas.

PATTERN II. The second pattern is presently found throughout North America, Western Europe, Australia, New Zealand, and many urban areas in Latin America. It is characterized by the likely origin and extensive spread of the HIV during the late-1970s. Most cases occur among homosexual and bisexual males and intravenous drug users (Torrey, Way, and Rowe 1988). Heterosexual transmission, representing a small percentage of cases, is increasing. Blood products for transfusion are screened and essentially safe. Perinatal transmission, from mother to child, is uncommon because of the relatively few women thus far infected.

PATTERN III. The third pattern is presently distributed in Eastern Europe, the Middle East, North Africa, and most countries of Asia and Oceania. Here, HIV infection appears to have been introduced relatively recently—during the early to mid-1980s. Currently these countries account for only a small percentage of AIDS cases, less than 1 percent of the reported total. Early infections as well as large percentages of people developing AIDS are generally associated with transfusions of blood products from other areas, especially Pattern I countries. An additional source of infection appears to derive from sexual contact with populations from Pattern I and II countries, and prostitutes are among the highest risk groups. It should be noted that these patterns are broad generalizations and different patterns may coexist within a single country, or even within a single large metropolitan area. Additionally, the patterns can be expected to change as the infection spreads through the populations of these countries (Mann 1988).

Though certainly not excluding any single country or region from consideration, these global patterns suggest that our focus be directed away from Pattern III countries and that we should concentrate our efforts on countries reflecting Patterns I and II characteristics. And indeed attention has been directed toward selected countries and regions within Patterns I and II, namely Haiti, Euro-America, and equatorial Africa.

The Haitian Context

In 1981, practically coincident with the report of the first cases of AIDS among the male homosexual community in the United States were reports of thirty-four cases of AIDS among Haitian immigrants to the United States and twelve cases of a disease previously unrecognized in Haiti, Kaposi's sarcoma, a soft tissue cancer and one of the opportunistic diseases indicative of AIDS (Barry, Mellors, and Bia 1984). Moreover, AIDS was identified among both Haitian men and women, and the men were reportedly not homosexual. Quite naturally, in addition to the attention directed toward the United States, Haiti was identified as a potential index location for the HIV, and several rather disparate cases have been made for a Haitian origin of HIV (figure 2.2).

Mentioned earlier, one historical scenario traces the origin of HIV to the travels of Christopher Columbus (Andre 1987). In addition to news of the discovery of a "new world," it is conjectured that Columbus's crew also brought back to Europe from Hispaniola (Haiti) a very contagious and "terrifying" disease manifest by cutaneous lesions, a deterioration of the general

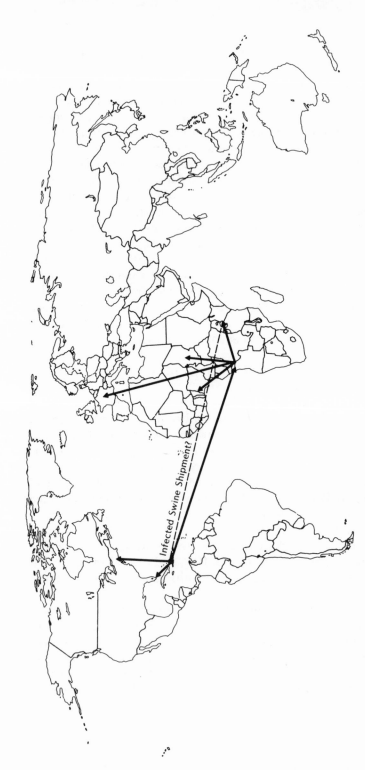

Figure 2.2. The Theory of Haitian HIV Origin

Infected Swine Shipment?

state, and "amputation of the genitals." Traditionally, this information has served as a basis for the "Columbian" or "American"
theory of the introduction of venereal syphilis into Europe and
the subsequent pandemic of the late fifteenth and early sixteenth centuries.

A second Haitian scenario involves the spread of the HIV or
its predecessor to human hosts in Haiti, as well as in equatorial
Africa, through the regular ingestion of uncooked animal blood
sacrificed in spirit-possession ceremonies (Moore and LeBaron
1986). In this case, the focus is directed toward Haiti rather than
equatorial Africa since the subsequent spread of the epidemic to
Western populations—the United States—was believed to occur
through international gay tourism to Haiti.

Though Haiti is nominally and ostensibly Roman Catholic,
it has been suggested that the large majority of Haitians partici-
pate in the voodoo cult, a religion with a pantheon of gods
derived in large part from Dahomey in West Africa. Spirit
possession of priests is an essential element of the voodoo religion. In Haiti, the spirits of the gods are summoned by the blood
sacrifice of bulls, goats, pigs, pigeons, and most commonly
chickens. If accurately described, the priests, in some type of
trance and possessed by a patron spirit, cut the throats of the
animals or, in the case of chickens, tear off their heads. The
priest may ingest the blood directly or the blood sacrifice may be
collected in a "gourd containing salt, ash, molasses, ornative
rum" (Moore and LeBaron 1986). This mixture is stirred and
allowed to coagulate, and then the priest and his other assistants ingest a portion. Also, in curing ceremonies, the blood
from the sacrificed animal may be rubbed on or into a patient's
afflicted part. Certainly, this practice provides frequent opportunities for exposure to animal blood that may contain a precursor to the HIV virus or possibly the HIV virus itself.

This religious practice is in turn connected with a reported
high incidence of homosexuality, or at least bisexuality, among
the male voodoo priests and their assistants (Metraux 1972).
Moreover, historical accounts of Haitian culture depict the attitude toward homosexuality as "one of derision rather than
vindictiveness," and male homosexuality is present in both the
cities and countryside (Herskovits 1971).

The next sequence in this theory involves homosexual contact between Haitians and tourists from North America and the high level of sexual activity among the latter during a period of the "gay liberation movement" (Leibowitch 1985; Moore and LeBaron 1986). More specifically, in the 1970s, Port-au-Prince developed as a popular resort area for homosexual men from the United States. Given the documented high incidence of multiple sexual partners among some homosexual men, it is hypothesized that the infection could have spread very rapidly to the tourists and, in turn, to the tourists' homosexual contacts upon their return to the United States.

Further, it is proposed that the infection traveled from Haiti to central Africa, most notably to Zaire, formerly the Belgian Congo. Without adequate preparation, Belgium granted independence to Zaire in the 1960s. The official language of the Belgian Congo was French, and to staff the civil service and administrative posts left vacant by the departure of the Belgians, Zaire recruited several thousand French-speaking Haitians. It is assumed the Haitians brought the HIV infection with them. From Zaire, the infection spread across central Africa and to Europe—to the latter by black Africans as well as white Europeans with strong ties to central Africa, and by Haitians who migrated to Belgium and France.

In summary, the Haitian scenario involves (1) the presence of HIV-related viruses in animals (possibly spread from African animals to those of the Caribbean), (2) the use of these animals in blood sacrifices associated with the voodoo religion, (3) direct ingestion of this blood by "houngans" or voodoo priests, (4) the practice of homosexuality by priests and the tolerance of homosexuality and its practice among the general male population, (5) development of Port-au-Prince as a resort for male homosexuals from the United States, (6) high levels of sexual activity among some male homosexuals, (7) the migration of Haitians to central Africa, and (8) the migration of black Africans and Haitians from central Africa to Belgium and France.

Haiti is not without its defenders. Some suggest that the "disproportionate" number of Haitians diagnosed as having AIDS may be owing to the intense surveillance of a "captive" population such as Haitian refugees in the United States. It is also suggested that the "outbreak" of AIDS in Haiti may have been magnified by the opportunistic infections and generally widespread immunosuppression among Haitians, resulting from chronic protein-calorie deprivation endemic on the island (Barry, Mellors, and Bia 1984). And some cite the difficulty in documenting risk factors such as homosexuality, sexual promiscuity, and drug abuse, the latter two illegal under the current Haitian government (Leonidas and Hyppolite 1983; Smith 1983). In this same area, some suggest the virus was introduced into the Caribbean from the United States by the homosexual and bisexual community (Aubry 1989).

Still other evidence has been presented against a Haitian origin for the HIV: (1) the recent appearance of Kaposi's sarcoma (KS) in Haiti, (2) previous homosexual and heterosexual contact between Haitians and foreigners without complication, and (3) lack of involvement of hemophiliacs in the United States prior to 1975. The latter argument is especially interesting.

Hemophiliacs require repeated transfusions of coagulant factor VIII derived from plasma. From around 1970, "concentrates" of this factor were used in the United States, derived from the mixed plasma of from 2,000 to 20,000 donors. It is now documented that, prior to 1980, there is no recorded trace of HIV infection or related conditions from any of the case records or autopsies of hemophiliacs. This is especially important to the Haitian hypothesis, since prior to 1975 much of the blood used in North America to develop the "concentrates" came from Latin America and the Caribbean, namely Haiti (Leibowitch 1985). After 1975, the Federal Food and Drug Administration would no longer grant approval to blood from Haiti or the majority of former South American suppliers. Therefore, one might conclude that, prior to 1976, Haitian donor/sellers were not carriers of the HIV.

Other information points to a recent development of the infection. A review of records of cancer biopsies from three private hospitals in Port-au-Prince with a combined total of 180 beds revealed no recorded cases of KS during the period from 1968 to 1983. And a review of 1,000 cancer biopsies at the Albert Schweitzer Hospital in Deschapelles, Haiti, during the same period also reveals no cases of KS. The earliest known patient with possible AIDS in Haiti appears to have been a young man who died in 1978 (Pape and Johnson 1989).

If, in fact, the virus was imported to Haiti, at least two sources of the infection are likely—namely, the United States and Africa.

A Euro-American Origin?

Despite the early identification of HIV-related conditions in the United States and the large numbers of reported AIDS cases in the United States and Western Europe, and recusing "the doctors of death" and bestiality hypotheses, there are currently few serious advocates of a Euro-American origin of HIV (figure 2.3).

In the very early phases of the epidemic, speculation centered on the United States and its male homosexual population. Indeed, the homosexual stamp was affixed to the disease: Gay Related Immune Deficiency (GRID). Attempts were made to link AIDS and AIDS Related Conditions (ARC) with some mutant immunosuppressor sperm, the result of homosexual hyperactivity (Leibowitch 1985). Of course, shortly thereafter, identification of AIDS and ARC in hemophiliacs, parenteral drug users, and other heterosexual individuals led to the discarding of this theory. And identification of ARC and AIDS in Haiti, central Africa, and Europe broadened geographic speculation on the origin of the disease agent.

Recusing bestiality, germ warfare, and some type of recombinant biological research accident as sources of HIV—all theories based on mere speculation—it is difficult to develop plausible mechanisms for the presence of HIV within humans or the transmission of an HIV precursor to humans from some animal reservoir within Europe or the United States. Some immediately dismiss the United States and Europe from consideration, suggesting it is impossible that AIDS conditions could have "broken out" in these regions on an epidemic scale before 1980 without having been noticed. Therefore, barring some major genetic mutation, it is improbable that the HIV was somehow created "on the spot."

Some who posit a Euro-American origin of HIV look to the morphologic and morphogenetic similarities between this virus

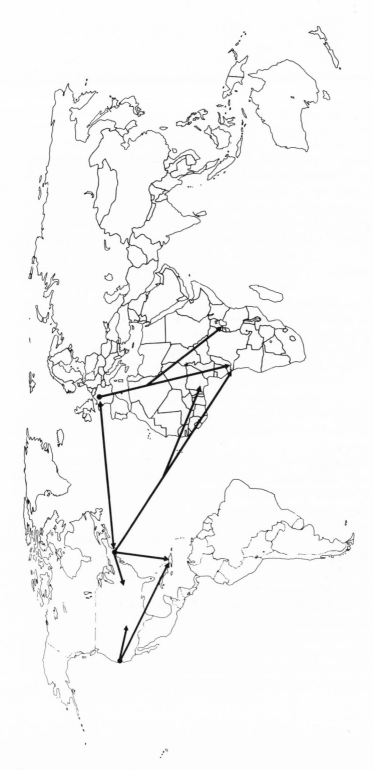

Figure 2.3. The Theory of Euro-American HIV Origin

and the visna-maedi virus found in sheep and goats (Najera, Herrera, and Andres 1987; Kantner and Pankey 1987). It has been proposed that the HIV is not a new virus and did not come from Africa but has been endemic in the "Euro-American" population since the beginning of the twentieth century. In one instance, "evidence" to support this endemicity includes some twenty-eight cases of disseminated Kaposi's sarcoma in Europe reported in the medical literature between 1902 and 1966.

How the virus spread to humans from these animal reservoirs poses an even greater problem to the authors of this hypothesis. They make but do not follow up on a statement that sexual contact between male humans and sheep has been documented, presumably implying that such contact was the mode of HIV transmission. Moreover, they discuss the formation of sadomasochistic clubs and an increase in traumatic sexual practices, again not explaining the linkages to the spread of the disease but suggesting that these sociocultural changes in society associated with the gay liberation movement caused the infection to become epidemic and to be exported somehow to Africa. Another source suggests that the HIV was exported to Africa in blood products from Europe and the United States (Sabatier 1987).

In one Euro-American origin scenario, (1) a virus closely related to the HIV was present in the sheep of northern Europe, (2) the virus was somehow transmitted to humans through human male sexual contact with the sheep, (3) the virus lay dormant for many years, (4) increased promiscuity and traumatic sexual practices developed among homosexuals in the 1970s, perhaps leading to mutation or a triggering of the virus, and (5) the HIV was transmitted to Africa in blood and blood products imported from Europe and the United States.

To date few comprehensive studies—and therefore little evidence in support of this Euro-American hypothesis—exist. Nevertheless, in some countries of Africa and Asia, the generally accepted view is that the HIV spread from Europe to Africa rather than the other way around or, coupled with anti-Western sentiment, that it began with American homosexuals and was spread around the world by American travelers and imported American blood products (Waite 1988; Sabatier 1987).

Out of Africa?

Attempts at retrospective identification of early HIV infection and AIDS cases in some countries of Africa as well as countries in other developed regions is problematic for a number of reasons (Hayes, Marlink, and Hardarvi 1989): (1) because resources are extremely limited, clinical record-keeping retains a low priority, (2) where there is clinical evidence suggestive of HIV infection or AIDS, the necessary corroborative laboratory evidence may be lacking, (3) the lack of resources may not permit diagnosis of AIDS by means of invasive techniques used in developed countries, and (4) immunologic testing of fresh and stored sera is difficult. False-positive confirmation tests by Western blot from fresh sera—the initial test used to detect antibodies to the HIV—have been reported, and the findings indicate that cross-reacting retroviruses may be circulating in tropical regions of Africa and other regions (Quinn and Mann 1989). Some older sera show immunologic reactivity despite the absence of HIV. It is probable that the Enzyme Linked Immuno Sorbent Assay (ELISA) testing yields a significant number of false positives, especially in areas of endemic malaria. Ideally, more specific tests are needed to confirm all repeatedly positive ELISA tests.

Amidst these problems and caveats, as well as continued published claims of a conspiracy among scientists and the media against Africa and persistent denials of the existence of a major health problem, several lines of evidence suggest that HIV-1 may have originated in eastern or central sub-Saharan Africa (Konotey-Ahulu 1987; Farthing, Brown, and Staughton 1988; Chiodi et al. 1989; Hayes, Malink and Hardarvi 1989; Essex 1989). The eastern and central regions of sub-Saharan Africa (figure 2.4), seven countries in particular, are important in this regard because of their proximity to the epicenter of the African AIDS outbreak and because of their relatively high reported incidence of AIDS. These countries include Burundi, Kenya, Rwanda, Tanzania, Uganda, Zaire, and Zambia (Yeager 1988).

Using more refined and reliable assays and Western blot criteria, corroborated sero-epidemiological and sero-archeological studies indicate the presence of HIV-1 infection in Africa

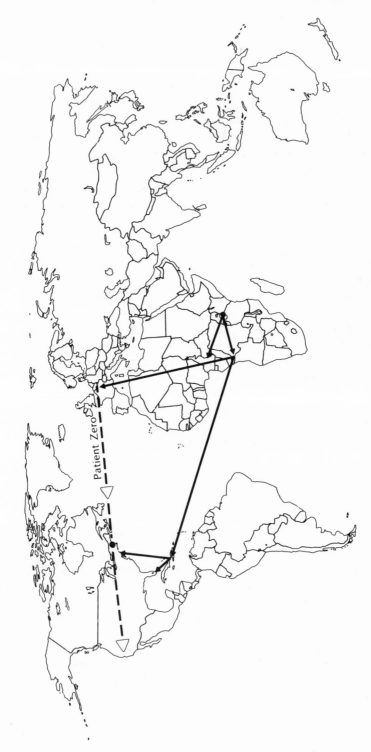

Figure 2.4. The Theory of African HIV Origin

as early as 1959 in a serum sample collected from Leopoldville, Belgian Congo, now Kinshasa, Zaire (Nahmias et al. 1986; Chiodi et al. 1989). In 1970 a pregnant woman was found to be HIV-1 seropositive in Kinshasa (Brun-Vezinet et al. 1984). Clinical records also indicate a suspected case of AIDS in a Danish surgeon apparently exposed to HIV-1 in Zaire between 1972 and 1975 (Bygbjerg 1983). Examination of sera collected in a northern Zairian equatorial region during investigations of an Ebola River fever outbreak indicates the presence of the HIV-1. Additionally, an isolate of HIV-1 was recovered from the serum of one antibody-positive person who subsequently died of an AIDS-like illness in 1978 (Nzilambi et al. 1988). Finally, a recent study of sera collected from several remote tribes in Zimbabwe, Liberia, and Kenya in the late 1960s and early 1970s confirmed the presence of HIV-1 in two specimens from the Mano tribe of Liberia (Chiodi et al. 1989). With the possibility of one exception (Garry et al. 1988), no serum samples stored in the United States prior to the 1970s have been found to be seropositive.

On the basis of these and other serological studies, there is some indication that HIV infection may have emerged earlier in Africa than in the United States. However, the rapidly rising incidence of cases in Africa also suggests a new epidemic of infection, perhaps as recent as forty to fifty years ago (Farthing, Brown, and Staughton 1988; Essex 1989; McClure and Schulz 1989).

One hypothesis suggests a primate reservoir of a precursor of HIV, the African green monkey. African green monkeys captured in the wild have a very high incidence, approximately 60 percent, of infection with an immunodeficiency virus closely related to HIV called Simian T-Lymphotropic Virus type III or Simian Immunodeficiency Virus (SIV) (Farthing, Brown, and Staughton 1988). This virus does not appear to cause AIDS in the African green monkey, but when injected into Asian macaque monkeys from a different continent it results in AIDS-like diseases and conditions.

However, it should be noted that the SIV is much more closely related to a second more recently discovered strain of HIV, namely HIV-2, than it is to HIV-1 (Essex 1989). The HIV-2 has been located in several countries of western Africa including

Cape Verde, Burkina Faso, Ivory Coast, Guinea-Bissau, and Senegal (Kanki, Alroy, and Essex 1985; Kanki et al. 1986; Clavel, Mansinho, and Chamanet 1987; Horsburgh and Homberg 1988; Essex 1989). It is reported that the class of reactivity seen with serum samples from West African prostitutes was virtually indistinguishable from that seen with serum samples from African green monkeys.

Since HIV-2 and SIV-1 seem highly related to each other and HIV-2 is apparently restricted to West African people, whereas SIV is present in green monkeys throughout much of Africa, the possibility that this virus moved from monkeys to people can obviously be considered. SIV, HIV-2, and HIV-1 are clearly related, and each is more closely related to one another than to other lentiviruses and the human retroviruses HTLV-1 and HTLV-2.

In any event, it seems less likely that an SIV in African green monkeys was the immediate precursor of HIV-1 but more likely that one did give rise to HIV-2. One hypothesis might be that HIV-1 moved into humans from a precursor virus in another as yet unidentified species.

With regard to the etiological origin of HIV infection among humans, therefore, the most cogent issues derive from the isolation of SIV from the African green monkey. Several tentative hypotheses have been posited to explain the possible route of transmission from monkeys to humans, including insect vectors such as mosquitoes, monkey bites, or the consumption of monkey meat.

Given the historical epidemiological experience of diseases such as yellow fever, malaria, and the plague, perhaps the most intuitively plausible thesis is the possibility of transmission of the pathogen by biting insects (Zuckerman 1986). Although it has been demonstrated that the HIV-1 can survive from several hours to days in insects fed or injected with blood containing high concentrations of HIV-1 (Lyons, Schoub, and McGillivray 1985), epidemiological evidence from Africa as well as the United States weighs heavily against the role of a blood-sucking arthropod as a vector. HIV-1 infection is rare in children, otherwise known to be risk-free, who are normally bitten most frequently by mosquitoes, fleas, lice, and the like. Also, no significant correlation between the presence of HIV-1 antibodies in humans and arboviruses in high incidence areas has been established (Biggar et al. 1985; Mann 1987; Castro et al. 1988). Furthermore, the concentration of HIV-1 in the blood of infected humans is quite low, further reducing the likelihood of transfer by biting insects.

Regarding the consumption of monkey meat, there is no substantive evidence to support the spread of the HIV-1 via the enteric route. And the relatively low concentration of HIV-1 in saliva renders the bite of an infected monkey quite an inefficient route of HIV transmission.

Certainly the possible origin of HIV in humans, whether HIV-1 or 2, remains in dispute (Essex and Kanki 1988; Mulder 1988), and no scientifically proven model exists for the method of transfer. Nevertheless, there are apparently extant certain practices in Africa that could bring humans in direct contact with blood from monkeys. Interestingly, one such practice has been documented among natives living in remote central Africa near the presumed epicenter of the African epidemic. In documenting the sexual customs and culture of people living in the Great Lakes region of central Africa in 1973, Kashamura (1973, 137) describes one practice of the Idjwi, who reside on an island in Lake Kivu between the borders of Rwanda and Zaire: "Pour stimuler un homme ou une femme et provoquer chez eux une activite sexualle intense, on leur inocule dans les cuisses, la region du pubis et le dos du san preleve sur un singe, pour un homme, sur un guenon, pour ne femme." (To stimulate a man or a woman and induce in them intense sexual activity, monkey blood (for a man) or female-monkey blood (for a woman) was directly inoculated in the pubic area and also in the thighs and back.)

If this description is accurate, the practice described would constitute a very efficient means of transferring the SIV to both males and females. And through genetic mutation, such a transfer could be in part responsible for the emergence of HIV-1 and HIV-2 in humans. It might also serve to corroborate a model that suggests that HIV infection may have existed and remained stable in remote areas of central Africa for a long period of time (Nzilambi et al. 1988). Further support for the long-standing presence of HIV infection among natives in remote areas derives from recent evidence of HIV-1 infection among the Sangha pygmy group in the isolated ecosystem of the Central African Republic (Gonzalez et al. 1987) and the first cases of AIDS in Uganda occurring among several businessmen who died at an isolated fishing village on Lake Victoria (Okware 1987).

In any event, the African origin scenario couples the diffusion of the infection on the continent with the corresponding period of rapid urbanization and international trade, specifically migrant labor systems, with the migration of young men to cities, and with the development of the infection in and the mobility of prostitutes. Of particular importance in this scenario is the Trans-Africa Highway, which is proposed to link Mombassa, Kenya, on the east coast to Lagos, Nigeria, on the west coast. Though far from completed, this road passes through Kenya, Uganda, and Rwanda (near Lake Kivu) to northern Zaire, the Central African Republic, Cameroon, and Nigeria. Reports from within Africa suggest that the HIV-1 infection appears to be spreading eastward from central Africa along the Trans-Africa Highway (Okware 1987).

If the initial reservoir of HIV infection is central Africa, several geographical pathways out of Africa have been suggested. Some countries of Western Europe have long established colonial ties with Africa and substantial concentrations of central African immigrants. For example, an estimated 6,000 to 8,000 residents from central Africa, mostly from Zaire, reside in Belgium (Clumeck et al. 1984). Many frequently return to Zaire for family or business purposes while others come to Europe for medical care. In fact, clinicians in Belgium and France particularly recognized a similarity between the description of AIDS cases from the United States in 1981 and patients arriving for medical evaluation from the central region of Africa (Biggar 1987). Also, some early cases of ARC and AIDS in France occurred among immigrants recently arrived from central Africa (Brunet, Boubet, and Leibowitch 1983; Ellrodt et al. 1984).

In this scenario, rather than moving from Haiti to Zaire, the Haitians recruited to fill civil service posts in the immediate post-independence period acquired the infection in Zaire and carried the infection with them as they returned to Haiti as well as to Europe (De Perre et al. 1984). Subsequently, primarily through international travel of homosexuals, the infection traveled from Haiti and possibly Europe to the United States. In turn, the United States and Europe served as reservoirs for further diffusion of the virus to other countries of the world.

    In summary, the African Origin Theory involves (1) the presence of HIV-precursors in the primate population throughout most of central Africa, (2) transmission of this precursor from an animal to a human host, (3) diffusion throughout central Africa supported by rapid urbanization, migration, and transcontinental transport, (4) diffusion to Haiti by Haitians returning from employment in Zaire, (5) diffusion to Europe via migrating black Africans and Haitians from central Africa, (6) infection of male homosexuals from the United States visiting Haiti, and (7) infection of populations in other countries by visiting Americans or the importation of infected blood products.

Several issues have been raised regarding the accuracy of the African Origin Theory. While some difficulties can be dismissed rather readily, others warrant close consideration. For example, if the AIDS epidemic resulting from HIV-1-infection were the outcome of transmission from monkeys, it is puzzling that it has not been possible to document infections with HIV-2 or other SIV-like viruses among populations within central Africa (Kitchen 1987). The widespread distribution of African green monkeys throughout equatorial African countries, the close relationships between HIV-2 and SIV, and the absence of HIV-2 from East-central Africa, the purported epicenter of HIV-1 infection, are particularly puzzling.

Recent evidence indicates that extensive genetic variation of SIV exists in African green monkeys from a single geographic region (Li et al. 1989). This extensive diversity justifies a continued search for isolates more closely related to HIV-1 and HIV-2, which would provide evidence for cross-species transmission between African green monkeys and humans as the origin of HIV syndrome viruses.

Another argument against the African origin of HIV asks, if Africa is the source of the infection, why was the syndrome first identified in American homosexuals and not in Africa? In part, the answer to this question may be related to the lack of appropriate diagnostic facilities in Africa to detect an emerging syndrome as polymorphous as HIV-related disease. Also, the early recognition of cases in the United States was possible partly because the virus was concentrated in limited groups at risk and was not spread over the general population, unlike the case in Africa (Desmyter et al. 1986).

Which Theory is Correct?

To date, there exists no conclusive scientific evidence for locating the exact origin of the HIV. As we have seen, the search for the origins of HIV has exhibited an unusual propensity to exacerbate existing tensions within the body politic (Sabatier 1987). Amidst claims and counterclaims, for example, efforts of Western researchers to locate the origins of HIV in Africa have been denounced as a conspiracy and perpetuation of racially motivated stereotypes. Tensions exist even within Africa. Some Nigerian athletes reportedly refused to attend the All-Africa Games in Nairobi, Kenya, because of the prevalence of AIDS there (Schmidt 1988). Certainly, caution must be exercised when interpreting data on HIV infection from any location.

What the search for possible origins of HIV indicates to me as a social scientist is that, regardless of geographic region, we are woefully lacking in our understanding of behavior patterns important to the transmission of HIV. Our knowledge of sexual practices appears to be as lacking and fragmented for the United States as it is for Zaire and Haiti. For example, we do not have accurate data on geographic variations in intranational and international homosexual practices. Legal sanctions against homosexuality in some countries and social sanctions in others certainly affect the accuracy of informants' responses to any such inquiries.

Similarly, we do not have accurate information on the sexual practices of heterosexuals, regardless of geographic location. If, as reported, anal intercourse is a particularly efficient means of transmitting the virus, it would seem essential to understand the incidence of this sexual practice among heterosexuals as well as homosexuals. Transmission of the virus via oral sex had been suggested several years ago, and a case study described recently appears to support the efficacy of this pathway (Spitzer and Weiver 1989).

HIV infection is spread through different types of behavior, and presently the best hope for stopping the epidemic is through changing the types of behavior responsible for its continued transmission. Yet human behavior and the forces that shape this behavior are among the most complex and poorly understood dimensions of this problem. The knowledge base in the behavioral and social sciences necessary for a search for the origins and spread of HIV is rudimentary at best.

Therefore, it is incumbent upon social scientists to establish the necessary knowledge base. It is also obvious that the various social sciences (and medical sciences) cannot work toward this goal in "splendid" isolation. The problem is too complex, and we do not have the luxury of unlimited amounts of time. It is time for increased cooperative and consolidated efforts within the social sciences, between anthropologists, geographers, psychologists, sociologists, and others, between social and medical scientists, and between both groups and representatives of persons living with HIV infection.

Perhaps reflecting my bias as a geographer, I would suggest further that the search for the origins of HIV as well as efforts to develop strategies to modify related behavior patterns proceed on a regional basis. The regional tradition is well established and continues to be strong in area studies, anthropology, and geography. We should build on these traditions and develop regionally specific research teams in cooperation with regional governments adequate to conduct the necessary sociobehavioral research.

3

Modeling the Geographic Spread of AIDS for Educational Intervention

PETER GOULD

In the AIDS epidemic, we are finally realizing that we face a new plague of global proportions (Gould 1969). As of January 1991, 157 countries had reported the presence of AIDS, and we believe that the Human Immunodeficiency Virus (HIV) is virtually everywhere. In some countries the consequences are already catastrophic and getting worse each year. In southwest Uganda, in the province of Kisii alone, there are already over 20,000 orphaned children from young parents who have died of AIDS, and the numbers have been nearly doubling for the past few years. Over 146,000 people in the United States have been diagnosed with full-blown AIDS, over half have already died, and we have no idea what the ultimate consequences may be because only now, ten years into the epidemic, are we slowly beginning to put together a picture of the rate of HIV infection in the general population.

Many of these basic numerical facts, numbers growing rapidly each day, are well-known to readers of this book, and I shall not spend much time on them in a simple account. Rather, I would like to point to an enormous void in our knowledge about the epidemic—a void illuminated by the geographic perspective, and the distinct understanding it brings for scientific, educational, and planning purposes. This is the first epidemic in modern history for which we have virtually no idea of its extent in geographic space, and as a result it appears literally "distant" and remote to most people. Many people consider AIDS essentially a disease of homosexuals and intravenous drug users . . . I'm not a homosexual, I'm not a drug user . . . why should I worry? AIDS is something that happens to other people at other places . . . it is not going to happen to me. But we now know that HIV is in at least 98 percent of the 3,300 counties in this country. We also know that there was a 40 percent increase in AIDS in the teenage population over the past two years, generally split between young men and women. The rate is one *percent* (not per thousand) in 15-16-year-olds in New York and Miami, and 2-3 *percent* in 21-year-olds. For runaway teenagers, seropositivity is 7 percent. Of more than 100,000 males with AIDS, 20 percent are in the low twenties, virtually ensuring that they were infected as teenagers, given the median time to conversion of 10 years.

Why is there this huge void in understanding and perception? In the United States and certainly some European countries, part of the ignorance is a result of the confidentiality issue, the idea that individuals with AIDS should not be identified except to fully qualified medical personnel. It is argued that geographic location of people with AIDS, specified by a very fine coordinate system or street address, could become an identifier. I believe this would be wrong, for perfectly understood ethical reasons. In all the mathematical modeling (the implications of which I shall discuss later), geographers have not identified anyone, have no need to identify anyone, and would not know what to do with such information if they had it. The loss of individual confidentiality is a genuine fear, but it has been taken to extreme and absurd lengths (Openshaw et al. 1989), so extreme and absurd that a vital component of our understanding is now in total disarray. In the United States, the Centers for Disease Control report only by state—Texas, California, etc.—a geographic scale so huge that it is analytically useless. It is also scientifically ridiculous: Rhode Island fits into Texas about 250 times. We now have published maps at the census tract level of a few blocks, and anyone with an ounce of intelligence, rather than a pound of bureaucratic stupidity, can see that no one could possibly identify an individual at this scale, roughly six orders of spatial magnitude below the state levels reported. In Europe it is the same story: Sweden, for example, reports the incidence of AIDS for Stockholm, Göteborg, Malmö, and "Other" in a country over 1,500 kilometers in length. *Where* the disease is is disguised very nicely.

But the lack of geographic understanding is also symptomatic of a larger geographic blindness that runs through our society, even to professional epidemiologists. I have spoken to Ph.D.s in epidemiology who never had even an introductory course in spatial modeling in their entire university careers and did not know of its existence. All thinking runs down the time line, and few think to ask where the numbers might be in geographic space. They have been stuck at top dead center since 1939, with Nigel Bailey's classic book on modeling epidemics through differential equations (Bailey 1975). In the mathematical modeling group of a conference sponsored by the Office of Science and Technology I attended in July 1989, one distinguished mathematician thought "spatial modeling" meant running around from Alabama to Wyoming applying a differential equation here, there, and everywhere.

There are really two traditions of mathematical modeling in epidemiology, both concerned exclusively with the temporal dimension. First, there is a statistical tradition that tries to extrapolate forward but finds that the bands of confidence widen so quickly into the future that not much can be said. One English epidemiologist at the White House Conference noted that by 1992 we can be 95 percent sure that there will be between 750 and 25,000 AIDS cases in Britain, but one wonders whether a model is really necessary to make such a statement. One doctor at the conference, a man who had been at the forefront of AIDS care in a San Francisco hospital from the beginning, said, "Who needs this modeling? I can extrapolate just as well with a plastic drawing curve!" Nevertheless, this statistical tradition has done valuable "backcasting," retrospectively modeling the early years of the epidemic about which we know very little (Brookmeyer and Gail 1986; Gail and Brookmeyer 1988). After all, the class of retroviruses was only discovered in 1977, and the HIV itself in the early 1980s, although we now know that the first cases in Europe (Denmark and Norway) go back to the late 1960s, always with an "African connection" (Froland et al. 1988; Shilts 1988).

The second tradition is the mathematical—essentially differential equations. In the United States, this tradition is trying to divide the population into finer and finer units—young, old, male, female, black, white, homosexual, bisexual, heterosexual, hemophiliac, etc.—so the number and size of the equations grow, requiring more and more estimations of intra- and inter-transmission rates, rates that are changing even as they are measured. For example, the rate of *new* infection in the San Francisco homosexual community in 1989 and 1990 was practically zero; in 1984 it was 19 percent (Keeling 1989). But rather than mathematizing, let us think instead: how do you estimate the transmission rate of HIV from black intravenous drug-using heterosexual teenagers to old Hispanic bisexual men? Well, say the differential modelers, the social and behavioral scientists will have to give us the rates. In the meantime, we will take the first eigenvalue of the Jacobian, and if it is greater than one, we know the epidemic will spread. Or did we know this already, without this massive and totally inappropriate mathematical apparatus? I think you can see how this tradition, which is undoubtedly powerful and dominant at the moment in the research "corridors of power," can quickly deteriorate into silly computer games of nonlinear systems. We must do more than create just another sandbox for scholars to play in at the expense of the public. We have got to do better than this, and that means breaking habits of thought that are tied exclusively to the historical or temporal domain. To *understand* the epidemic, we must think about it in both space and time. We have all got to be geographers. Predicting the next number coming to us out of the future is not enough: we must predict the next map or maps, not simply for educational intervention, as we shall see, but as inputs to spatial assignment and allocation problems of always scarce medical resources. With 392,000 AIDS cases predicted by 1992, we know that new hospices and medical centers for terminally ill people must be close to them, must be properly allocated in geographic space. This is a rich and well-developed area of analytical geography over the past quarter of a century, and for all practical purposes we have algorithms to solve any variation on the basic spatial assignment theme.

Before considering two case studies for which the mathematical modeling is tied to the requirements of educational intervention, let us consider briefly the situation in Africa as a part of the global situation. We do have a global model that has worked quite well for predicting the spread of influenza to the world's largest fifty-one cities (Longini, Fine, and Thacker 1986; Rvachev and Longini 1985), and the same "connectivity structure," based on airline data, has been used by Flahault and Valleron (1989) in Paris to simulate the spread of AIDS with various "origin points" such as San Francisco, Casablanca, Nairobi, and Bangkok. Only an origin at Nairobi produces a map that bears a reasonable resemblance to the current global intensities.

The current situation in Africa is indicative of the consequences that may occur when the AIDS epidemic gets totally out of hand. The situation in East Africa is catastrophic, based on a review I made early in 1989 for the World Health Organization (WHO) of 300 lines of seroprevalence data from Tanzania, Uganda, Rwanda, and Zaire. At the moment, 80-90 percent of the prostitutes test seropositive; well over 30 percent of the truck drivers are seropositive, and it is known that they are major carriers of the HIV all the way from Somalia to Zambia. More than two years ago, Cuban doctors established that 33 percent of the Ugandan army (not the most disciplined troops in the world) were seropositive, while over 20 percent of women coming in for prenatal care to Kampala hospitals are also HIV-infected. Along the northwestern shore of Lake Victoria, an area previously plundered and pillaged by Idi Amin's troops, a mass migration-evacuation is taking place, ostensibly to escape from the epidemic. Other provinces will now experience a massive influx of HIV carriers. In some hospitals of Zaire, 20 percent or more of the medical staff (doctors and nurses) are infected, not through handling AIDS patients but through their own unprotected sexual relations. After reviewing such figures, I did not make myself particularly popular at WHO by telling them that most of the data were analytically useless.

An enormous amount of financial and medical resources has been devoted to tests and surveys, but there is very little you can do with the figures except hang them on the wall and look at them. In the entire country of Uganda, there are only two geographically specific points at which we know the rate of HIV infection in the general population, and these surveys have not been monitored and followed up. Most of the information is redundant in the literal information theoretic sense that it has no surprise value. What is the use of testing the prostitutes of Bongo when you know that at least 80 percent of them will be seropositive before you send yet another expensive medical team to do the testing?

It also appears highly likely that the hospitals themselves may be a major source of infection, since needles have to be used many times, and many hospitals do not have the facilities for proper sterilization. Transmission through blood transfusion has also been high. Similarly, and particularly tragic, the child immunization program is in disarray, not only from multiple needle use, but also because attenuated vaccines and inoculations may actually give a child another disease if his immune system is already down from HIV.

In West Africa the situation is rapidly approaching the seriousness of that in the East. In Abidjan, 60 percent of the patients at the university hospital, 10 percent of blood donors, 10 percent of pregnant women, and about half the prostitutes carried HIV. Abidjan has been called the "sexual crossroads" of Africa, something you can see by simply plotting air connections from every francophone country. A traffic of HIV needs a backcloth, a structure, to be transmitted. These air schedules and connections allow government ministers and their large entourages to attend "conferences" and have weekends of "rest and relaxation" at their taxpayers' expense. The result is that one-third of the blood samples from infected people in the Côte d'Ivoire are positive to both HIV-1 and HIV-2—in other words, both the East and West African varieties.

Under these conditions, with no cure or vaccine in sight, education is all we have. Yet one wonders how effective this can be under most African conditions: a landrover comes into a small rural village, two young bureaucrats "from the city" pass out pamphlets and harangue the people for ten minutes, and then they drive on to the next village. It is difficult to think this could be effective, but what alternative is there?

Education in Western Europe and North America can probably have a greater impact if it is undertaken frankly and forcefully. But it must be done quickly, and it should have started at least five years ago. AIDS is not something remote: it is literally all around us. Heterosexual transmission is growing month by month both absolutely and relatively, and while the homosexual community has shown radical changes in protective behavior, needle sharing is still a major route of transmission. And this is not just a problem of the drug community: a random survey of university athletes last year indicated that 30 percent had used steroids at some point (Keeling 1989), opening up another young and vital population to needle transmission. As for hemophiliacs, the fact is that there may be hardly any around in ten years. It takes hundreds of blood units to make one factor 8 clotting injection, and even with rigorous testing the probability of HIV getting through remains high when we consider the number of units required. For example, if testing lets only 1 in 1,000 infected samples through, then $1-(.999)^{200}$ still represents a probability of 0.18, or 18 percent chance, that a shot will be infected. In the early 1980s, the probability was close to 1.0 or certainty when the American blood industry, advised by the medical profession, said that HIV infection could not be passed via blood transfusion. For a number of years the industry refused to consider testing, saying it would be too expensive. It actually costs the American armed forces $4.31 to test a blood sample for HIV. As of August 1990, there were over 4,700 people with AIDS in the United States as a result of HIV-infected blood transfusions at time of surgery or blood coagulation shots for hemophilia.

In the absence of compulsory testing or a national survey, much of our understanding of the geographic extent of the epidemic in the United States comes from a continuing survey of young people (roughly 18-23 years old) volunteering for military service (Brundage et al. 1989). We now have over 2 million samples, by far the largest survey of anywhere in the world with the exception of Cuba, a country that was reported to have tested over 3 million of its citizens in 1988 and the rest by the end of 1989. Cuba is one of the countries that has undertaken quarantine of its 242 seropositives so far, mainly because it is determined not to have a catastrophic epidemic from soldiers returning from Angola.

Statisticians tend to denigrate the large military survey, saying that it is confined to a small age cohort and contains a great deal of self-selection. This is true, and it may be its greatest strength. Homosexuals, IV drug users, hemophiliacs, and those who suspect seropositivity and test before applying, do tend to self-select out, since they perceive the military as being antagonistic to their behavior. Thus, the county rates may well represent young and heterosexually dominant America. In 1989 these rates were between 0 and 10 per thousand, with a mean around 3 per thousand (Keeling 1989), approximately the same rate as that found by a recently completed national university survey. Many people's reaction is that this is quite small and nothing to worry about, but for a school the size of my own university, Penn State, with about 37,000 students at University Park, these figures mean that we have approximately 110 students who are HIV-positive, almost certainly ignorant of it, sexually active, and capable of spreading it to others.

The trouble is that many young people exhibit the well-known "immortality syndrome," the feeling that "it can't happen to me" (Brooks-Gunn, Boyer, and Hein 1988). Large surveys of teenagers in Massachusetts and Ohio have shown that few exhibited any anxieties about the spread of AIDS. And while a three-year longitudinal study of university students at Penn State showed a steady change in protective behavior, 50 percent still used no latex condom barrier for fairly casual sexual relations (DiClemente, Zorn, and Femoskok 1986; Flora and Thorenson 1988; Koch and Peckman 1989; Moeller and Bachman 1988; Shafer 1988).We also know, from many studies in health education, that the simple provision of information is not enough to change behavior. There must be a perception of quite personal health risk before behavior changes (Sisk, Hewitt, and Metcalf 1988; Strunin and Hingson 1987; Young, Koch, and Preston in press), and professionals in health education speak of definite "cues to action." In brief, something has to be done to make the epidemic concrete, real, and personal, not simply something "out there," distant and remote from an individual's daily life. It is my contention that when people actually see the geographic dynamics of the epidemic, when they see it "all around them," they then begin to reflect carefully upon the possibility of their own personal danger.

Very few published maps are available showing the geographic details of the AIDS epidemic, although in the United States a generalized AIDS surface shows a highly peaked distribution typical of many human geographic phenomena. Yet even at this small scale we can still see a corridor effect all the way down the East Coast, from Boston to Miami, following I-95, one of the major interstate routes (Gould 1989). Regional studies of HIV diffusion, based on the large military surveys, also reflect the way in which the human structuring of geographic space "channels" the epidemic, and they disclose a quite classical wave-like diffusion from major epicenters (Brown 1981; Morrill 1968). All the regional examples display strong spatially contagious diffusion, and somewhat weaker hierarchical diffusion controlled by the structure of urban interactions (Berry 1972; Gould 1969). Both types, of course, are present in any epidemic today. The disease tends to jump down the urban hierarchy to form regional epicenters (Cliff et al. 1981), and from these the daily commuter traffic allows it to spread into the surrounding countryside.

We can see these effects quite clearly in the case of Ohio, where we are allowed to observe the epidemic through the spatio-temporal "window" of a county and a quarter. Ohio is one of several case studies we are using to model the epidemic via expansion (Casetti 1972, 1982, 1986), transformation (Gould, Gorr, and Casetti 1988), and spatial adaptive filtering methods (Foster and Gorr 1985, 1986; Gorr and Hsu 1985; Makridakis and Wheelwright 1977). This is not the place for a detailed, technical presentation: it is sufficient to say that we can predict the next map about 96 percent accurately, and so use these predictions in animated map sequences for television presentation and educational intervention. Unfortunately, we have not yet arrived at the age of animated books, and we shall have to rely on traditional black and white map sequences, rather than fully animated maps in color (Gould, DiBiase, and Kabel 1989). The map sequences (figures 3.1 and 3.2) have been taken from "stills" in the animations and have deliberately been left untouched for printed presentation. This rather bare and unconventional cartography makes the point that map animation opens up an entirely new frontier in graphical presentation, for there is no need for text when a voice is available to describe a very dramatic and animated sequence showing the spatial dynamics of the AIDS epidemic.

Furthermore, the loss of color is serious for the purpose of graphical rhetoric, using "rhetoric" in its old and honorable sense of the art of persuasion. After all, the animated sequences are created to reach out and persuade young people to reflect carefully, and in quite personal terms, about the dangers of the epidemic. In viewing the two sequences here, keep in mind that you are seeing the development of contoured "AIDS surfaces" based on 88 and 67 county control points, and that gray tones substitute for a spectrum of cool to warm colors. Moreover, the contour interval is geometric, rather than the arithmetic interval of the usual topographic map. Each change of gray tone (color) represents three times the value of the previous one.

The first AIDS case recorded in Ohio was in 1981 in Cleveland, and by 1982 it had jumped down the urban hierarchy to nearby Akron and Canton, and then to Columbus, the capital in the middle of the state (figure 3.1). Of course, we do not know if this actually happened. We are not allowed to observe individual patient records, and by this time they would probably not tell us much anyway. It is possible that the first AIDS case in Columbus was the result of a homosexual visit to New York or San Francisco, but we have no way of telling this. In this initial "seeding" stage of the epidemic, it is becoming increasingly clear that in-migration of infected cases may play an important role. But such uncertainty does point out the problem of "system closure": Ohio is highly connected to the rest of the American system, and the United States is by far the most highly connected national piece of the international structure.

By 1983, the spatially contagious "wine stain on a tablecloth" diffusion has continued around the original epicenter of Cleveland, and we can now see two other regional epicenters in Columbus and Cincinnati. One or two cases are also recorded elsewhere, but we do not know if these are the result of sexual or

Figure 3.1. The Diffusion of AIDS in Ohio, 1981-1987

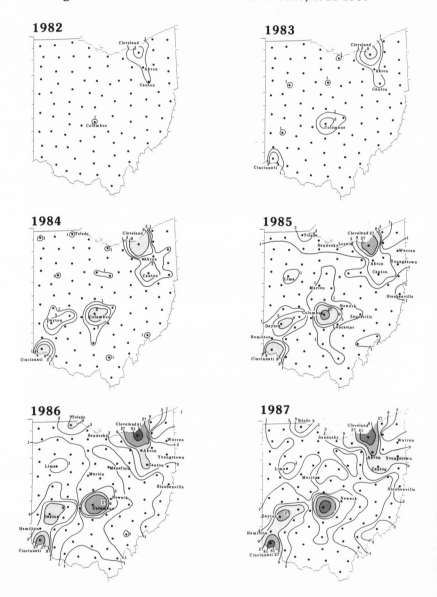

IV transmission. They could be the result of surgical transfusion or a hemophiliac injection.

By 1984, there is an intensification in the original regional epicenters, and we begin to get the first hint of a strong northeast-southwest alignment that follows a major corridor of high-speed road, rail, and air linkages. Since HIV is carried by one person to another, it is not surprising that basic geographic patterns of human spatial interaction appear as major corridors of infection.

By 1985, we see the diffusion moving outward from major epicenters, and the beginning of another alignment across the northern part of the state, again a major alignment of interstate highways linking secondary urban centers. By 1986, the three growing regional "amoebas" have linked together, and the uninfected rural areas are being squeezed smaller and smaller.

The process continues in 1987, the last year for which we had reliable data at the time the animated computer sequence was made. There are inevitable reporting delays, and in Ohio each case reported is carefully traced back to the county of residence rather than the place where the disease was diagnosed. Nevertheless, I think you will agree that we have seen a rather dramatic map sequence, in which you can feel, quite intuitively, a great deal of emerging spatio-temporal structure. It is rather like a photographic plate developing, with the final image faintly contained in the initial one. If I displayed all the maps in a row, and gave you a blank map for 1988, I think you would be able to make a fairly accurate, if intuitive, prediction of what will happen next. This is precisely what the mathematical modeling is about: we simply want to achieve a good mathematical description of the spatio-temporal structure, and use it to predict the next map or maps in the sequence.

This is the sequence we have in animated form on a computer display, and the impact has been great. A group of black teenagers from Florida visiting Penn State, young high school women, and university students who have seen the display all react in the same way. After the sequence was used on one program on public television, even the hardened and blasé television crew and cameramen said to me, "My God! We never realized it was that close."

Figure 3.2. The Diffusion of AIDS in Pennsylvania, 1981-1988

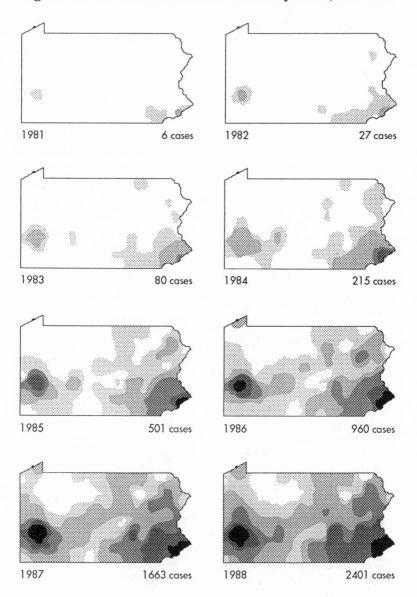

1981   6 cases

1982   27 cases

1983   80 cases

1984   215 cases

1985   501 cases

1986   960 cases

1987   1663 cases

1988   2401 cases

Finally, let us turn to Ohio's next-door neighbor, Pennsylvania, where the first case was also recorded in 1981. By the end of the year, six cases had been recorded (figure 3.2), and we can already see the emergence of what will become the major epicenter in Philadelphia in the southeastern corner of the state. Notice that a few of the cases are just to the west of Philadelphia, directly in alignment with the Pennsylvania Turnpike. Once again, the human structuring of geographic space is crucial for understanding the spread of HIV and AIDS, and we will see additional evidence in the pattern for later years. For example, by 1982 the westward movement from Philadelphia has increased, and one can see the first effects of the northeast turnpike extension. Meanwhile, the epidemic is increasing in the two major epicenters of Philadelphia, as well as in Pittsburgh, in the western part of the state.

In the following year we continue the "developing photographic plate" effect, and by 1984 one can see hierarchical effects as the epidemic jumps to Scranton and Harrisburg, north and west of Philadelphia. Meanwhile, spatially contagious effects are equally clear around the major and smaller epicenters. By 1985, another "channelling" effect in geographic space appears, this time east and northeast from Pittsburgh to Johnstown, and then following Route 220 to Altoona, State College, and Williamsport. The alignment is very clear by 1986, and by 1987 it is a distinct diagonal slash following the northeast-southwest alignment of the ridge-and-valley section of central Pennsylvania.

By 1988, there are only a few areas left untouched, and most of these are in the northern tier with national and state forests and very low population densities. Given the median time to conversion of ten years, this was probably the rough extent of HIV infection in 1978. There is evidence that the AIDS distributions reflect the HIV surfaces the decade before in rather the same way that lung cancer in women strongly matches the increases in women smoking after World War II.

Obviously, the map animation and mathematical modeling we have undertaken is not an academic exercise. These map sequences, including the predicted maps, have been made into a television tape that has been sent to the AIDS surveillance units of the fifty states and all the U.S. Public Health Service Regions to let them see how the geographical dynamics of the disease can be used in educational intervention campaigns (Gould, DiBiase, and Kabel 1989). All the experiences we have had to date indicate that these sequences have a very high visual impact, for many people start looking immediately for their own location to see how close the epidemic is to them. It is our hope that these visual materials, in the form of properly animated cartography, will provide precisely those "cues to action" that will make young people reflect very carefully about their own personal health risks in the future. In brief, this is what geographers mean by "bringing it home."

*Some of the materials of this essay were previously presented as "La diffusion du SIDA dans l'espace geographique" at the University of Lausanne and as "The Diffusion of AIDS in Geographic Space" at the Technical University of Zurich, May 1989.

4

Communities at Risk: The Social Epidemiology of AIDS in New York City

ERNEST DRUCKER

AIDS in New York City, 1981–1991

By the time this chapter appears in print, New York City will have reported over 35,000 cases of AIDS. With less than 3 percent of the nation's population, NYC accounts for almost 20 percent of all AIDS cases in the United States. Yet even this stark measure of the disproportionate impact of the epidemic on one locality understates both the extent and the character of the problem, for it is the devastating impact of AIDS on particular urban neighborhoods and communities that really distinguishes this phase of the epidemic in America.

AIDS, like most epidemics, is not best understood as a single outburst of infection or disease affecting an entire population or large geographic region with equal force. The Human Immunodeficiency Virus (HIV) is a blood-borne, sexually and perinatally transmitted infection. Its spread is based on the most intimate patterns of human contact. Accordingly, AIDS moves at different rates through different subpopulations, spreading as a function of the determinants of intimacy, largely social and geographic in nature. Populations at risk for AIDS are better defined by their social and behavioral characteristics than by any biological susceptibilities, although these are also important. Social class, race, age, and their association with the basic risks for transmission of HIV and AIDS (i.e., sexuality and drug use) form the context of this epidemic.

Further, in New York City and in other American cities, the very distinctive geographic patterning of these factors places many of its local communities at exceptionally high risk. Small-scale geographic differences in the prevalence of HIV are closely linked to those social and behavioral characteristics that determine the probable risk of infection for others in the same communities—even for those not in the original risk groups. These local patterns are essential for understanding and controlling the AIDS epidemic.

As the infection establishes itself in these high-risk groups and communities, it first deepens in each, producing endemic levels. We can see this in the high rates of infection within the specific well-established risk groups—gay men and IV drug users—and in the geographic concentration of these cases in certain neighborhoods of the city. Then, depending on each group or community's position in the larger social order (i.e., its sexual or drug-using contact with those outside), AIDS extends beyond these local communities to the city as a whole and, ultimately, to the wider population beyond the urban epicenter.

The dynamism of this process can be seen in the changing characteristics of AIDS cases reported in NYC over the last few years. These cases form the most visible face of the disease and are generally perceived as *the epidemic*. Individuals sick with full-blown AIDS are what we know most directly, and, in the aggregate, these cases have the most immediate impact on the community and its health care and social service systems. At first, it is the acceleration of the incidence of AIDS cases that is most dramatic. As table 4.1 shows, it took almost five years—from 1981 to 1985—for the first 5,000 AIDS cases to occur in NYC; the second 5,000 took only one and a half years, and the next 5,000 only fourteen months. In 1991, NYC expects over 10,000 new cases and 7,000-8,000 deaths (New York City Department of Health 1990).

This rapid growth in the incidence of AIDS cases sends shock waves through the communities most severely affected. Quickly people in these areas and risk groups come to know personally someone who is sick and, soon thereafter, several people. This phenomenon, which the sociologist Kai Erickson likens to a natural disaster, was seen first and most dramat-

Table 4.1. Known Mortality among Adult Cases by Period of Diagnosis, New York City

	No. of cases	Percent known dead[a]
1981 Jan.-June	40	90%
July-Dec.	100	93%
1982 Jan.-June	178	90%
July-Dec.	304	91%
1983 Jan.-June	461	90%
July-Dec.	533	91%
1984 Jan.-June	776	84%
July-Dec.	949	85%
1985 Jan.-June	1,233	83%
July-Dec.	1,423	82%
1986 Jan.-June	1,813	81%
July-Dec.	2,124	79%
1987 Jan.-June	2,393	72%
July-Dec.	2,426	65%
1988 Jan.-June	2,851	56%
July-Dec.	2,640	47%
1989 Jan.-June	2,351	31%
July-Dec.	1,705	10%
1990 Jan.	41	7%
Total[b]	24,383	
Total cumulative deaths	15,364	63%[c]

[a]Reporting of deaths is incomplete.   [b]Table totals include 42 cases diagnosed prior to 1981, 38 of whom are known to have died.   [c]1,929 additional death dates, identified through semiannual death certificate match, were added in this report.   Source: New York City Department of Health 1990.

ically in some of the gay communities of New York and San Francisco—for example, Fire Island and the Castro, where young gay men "buried" thirty or more friends in just a few years' time (Shilts 1988). A similar shockwave is also rapidly appearing in places like the Bronx. Figure 4.1 shows how, between 1982 and 1985, AIDS hospital admissions in the Bronx rose rapidly and clustered in the poorest areas of the South Bronx (Drucker 1986).

Figure 4.1. Hospital Admissions for Immune Disorders in the Bronx

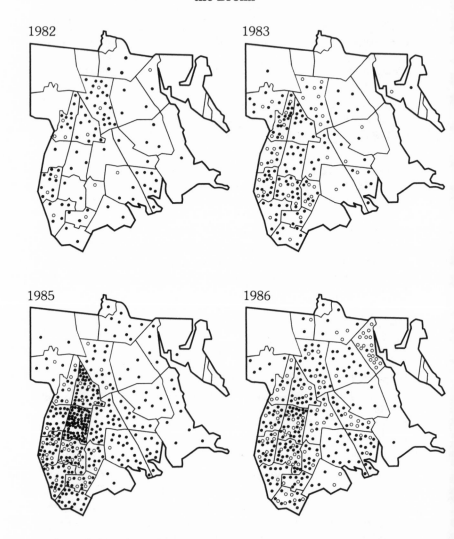

. One Male Admission
₀ One Female Admission

Source: New York State Department of Health

New York City, however, soon experienced another even more striking development in the pattern of AIDS cases, as the center of gravity of the epidemic began to shift away from the original dominant risk group of gay men. In August of 1988, for the first time in NYC, newly reported cases of AIDS among drug users and their sexual partners outnumbered those of homosexual and bisexual men (New York City Department of Health 1990). More cases of AIDS related to drug use also signified increased prevalence of AIDS among heterosexuals, African-Americans, Hispanics, and women and infants. These trends have continued since August 1988, and the difference widens with each month as an increasing proportion of cases are among drug users and their sexual partners.

Yet, even these appalling figures on AIDS cases and deaths do not paint the most accurate portrait of the epidemic's significance for the population of NYC. Ultimately, it is the underlying cause of AIDS—the HIV infection—that offers the most complete and revealing picture of both the current epidemic in the city and its probable future course. There is already a very large group of HIV-infected adults in NYC, estimated at 180,000-220,000 people (Health Systems Agency, 1989). The sheer size of this groups is central for assessing the impact of AIDS on NYC as a whole. And ultimately it is the uneven geographic and social distribution of this large population of HIV-infected people that determines the epidemic's powerful impact on many local communities. It does this first by affecting incidence—the rate of new HIV infections. Whether by sexual transmission, needle sharing, or pregnancy and childbirth, AIDS spread is ultimately driven by the background prevalence levels of HIV. Most infected individuals in NYC do not know their status; fewer than 10 percent have been tested positive. This group will, for many years, represent a substantial risk for transmission to others in New York, mostly through unprotected heterosexual intercourse and continued widespread IV drug use—both behaviors that are unlikely to change rapidly given our inability to discuss human sexuality openly or treat drug use as something other than a crime.

The second aspect of this early phase of the epidemic's course in NYC has to do with the rate of progression toward full-blown

AIDS and related symptomatic states of those individuals already infected. The long and variable latency of the virus, a median elapsed time of eight to ten years between infection and the appearance of full-blown AIDS (Hessol et al. 1989), plays a crucial role in interpreting HIV prevalence data. If the infection of HIV antedates the appearance of AIDS cases by almost ten years, the timing of the spread of the original epidemic of HIV infection and the age characteristics of those newly infected must be reinterpreted, both are pushed back. What we see as AIDS cases now are the result of a pattern of epidemic spread long past. This latency, which determines the timing of new cases of full-blown AIDS, also shapes the demand that the epidemic will place on a number of vital resources in the community, family support structures, health and social services, foster care, and housing all are affected today by HIV infections transmitted a decade or more ago. Even our most successful efforts at prevention or the development of a vaccine will not deter this element of AIDS impact on these communities.

AIDS in the Underclass

There are an estimated 200,000 IV drug users in NYC (Health Systems Agency 1989), 50 to 60 percent of them already infected with HIV (Des Jarlais et al. 1989). This large population of HIV-infected drug users are concentrated in New York's inner-city communities where their ethnic and racial composition, age, and social characteristics all have enormous significance for gauging the impact of AIDS on specific neighborhoods. And while IV drug users can be found in every social stratum and in every community (Eisenhandler and Drucker 1990), the very high prevalence of drug use among the poor and its association with specific risk behaviors needed for transmitting HIV (the sharing of syringes and needles, attendance at shooting galleries, and, most recently, the sex-for-crack phenomenon) are most often found in the inner-city communities.

This geographic focus of AIDS risk in specific NYC communities can be seen clearly in the distinctive distribution of even the earliest AIDS cases among the two largest risk groups—homosexual and bisexual men and IV drug users (figure 4.2)

Figure 4.2. Distribution of AIDS Cases in New York City, 1981-1984

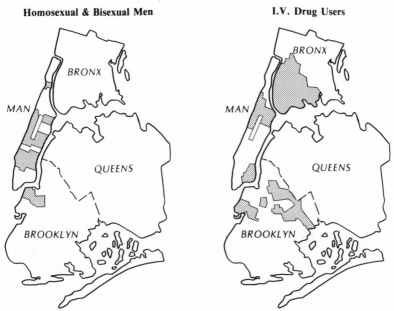

Homosexual & Bisexual Men   I.V. Drug Users

Source: Krystal, et al.1985. American Journal of Epidemiology

(New York City Department of Health AIDS Surveillance 1986). The geographic concentration of different populations with high rates of HIV has several important implications for the spread of infection. First, because of the high absolute rate of HIV infection among NYC's IV drug-using population (50-60 percent) and the high prevalence rates of drug use in many inner-city communities, the geographic concentration of drug use coincides with a geographic concentration of HIV-infected individuals. This produces very high rates of overall population prevalence in many discrete localities. For example, in the South Bronx (with a population of 500,000), 10-20 percent of the *entire population* of 25-45-year-old men are already infected, as are 5-8 percent of all women in the same age range (Drucker and Vermund 1989). At Bronx Lebanon Hospital in the heart of the area most hard hit, this projection is confirmed by reported rates of 5-10 percent among all women giving birth (Ernst 1990), and 14-25 percent of all emergency room admissions, and 25 percent of all non-AIDS in-patients (Centers for Disease Control 1990a). Other communities in NYC and in northern New Jersey appear to have comparable prevalence rates, levels which approximate those of some areas of East and central Africa.

The geographic patterning of HIV coincides with that of several other variables that are highly pertinent to understanding the AIDS epidemic in NYC. For example, the distribution of teenage pregnancy in NYC (the percentage of live births to women under 19 years of age) is as high as 27 percent in those same areas of the city with the highest rates of AIDS among IV drug users. And this geographic correspondence underscores the significance of the variable itself, clear evidence that early, unprotected sexual intercourse is a major risk factor for transmission of HIV.

While complete HIV population prevalence data are not generally available for NYC, AIDS case data can be used to model the probable distribution of HIV infection among the subpopulations of these communities. These data indicate a median age of AIDS cases at thirty-five years of age, with most HIV infections in the 25-45 age range. Back-calculating from these cases and utilizing the 8-10-year median latency of HIV infection suggests that transmission for this group took place in the early 1980s while most were in their early to mid-twenties. Thus in these areas, the teenage pregnancy data are precursory of heterosexual exposure to HIV, a pattern already evident in adolescent AIDS cases (Vermund et al 1989).

The geographic distribution of race/ethnicity are also quite specific in NYC. Among IV drug users and sexual partners with AIDS, about 85 percent are African-American or Hispanic—a pattern that is most powerfully evident in predicting pediatric AIDS cases, over 90 percent of which occur among minorities (New York City Department of Health, 1990). Figure 4.3 shows the geographic distribution of NYC communities with high proportions of African-American and Hispanic residents.

Even within the inner-city communities of NYC, both drug use and sexual contact patterns, with their attendant risk for transmission, are extremely local. "Shooting galleries" and crack houses are neighborhood institutions; drug "copping" and

Figure 4.3. Patterns of Segregation in New York City

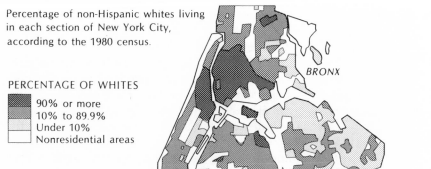

Percentage of non-Hispanic whites living in each section of New York City, according to the 1980 census.

PERCENTAGE OF WHITES

- 90% or more
- 10% to 89.9%
- Under 10%
- Nonresidential areas

BRONX

MAN.

QUEENS

BROOKLYN

sharing networks are usually based on teenage gang membership (itself usually bound to "turf") or social relations originating on the street corner in early adolescence, and in social clubs and party circuits. "The block" is still the basic geographic unit for urban drug sales territories (Williams 1989; Hamid 1990).

In addition to these neighborhood social structures affecting drug use, sexual contact patterns are also quite local in nature. And these patterns, probably more than drug use, are highly concordant by age, race, and ethnicity. In one study of over four hundred women receiving first trimester abortions at a South Bronx clinic (Drucker et al. 1989a), concordance with age, race, and ethnicity of sexual activity is apparent in the patterns of sexual contacts with men of the same race/ethnicity and, as sexually active women reach age 25, the likelihood of their sexual contact with those men in the age group most likely to be HIV infected (ages 25-45) increases (See table 4.2.)

This high risk for sexual exposure to HIV associated with the routine and characteristic age and ethnic patterns of sexual contact in this population is also reinforced by geography. In our study (Drucker et al. 1989a), almost 50 percent of these women's sexual partners came from the same postal zip code, generally within a few city blocks of the home of the woman interviewed. In such communities, high population prevalence levels of HIV among sexually active males can lead to chains of HIV infection that are sustained over long periods, irrespective of the fact that the original mode of transmission was needle sharing.

An early indication of this developing HIV endemicity in the inner city can be seen in the results of New York State's program of HIV testing for all newborns. In 1988, close to 2 percent of women delivering babies in the inner-city areas of New York were HIV-infected (Novick et al. 1989). Between one-third and one-half of these women lack any history of IV drug use themselves, and this proportion appears to be rising (Abrams 1990). In all likelihood, these women were themselves the sexual partners of previously-infected drug-using men. But, of course, even those women who *do* have histories of IV drug use were, almost universally, also the sexual partners of men (sometimes many men) who were IV drug users. Thus, it becomes extremely difficult to attribute these women's infection to one exposure or the other, since they were dually exposed for sustained periods of time to both risks for infection, indeed, the two risk factors are synergistic since frequent sexual exposure of women is sometimes linked to prostitution to obtain funds for drugs.

Women constitute the fastest growing group of new AIDS cases (Centers for Disease Control 1990a) but the percentage of women with AIDS differs dramatically by geographic region. While for the U.S. as a whole, fewer than 10 percent of AIDS cases are women, in the South Bronx, Harlem, and Newark, over 25 percent are female (New York City Department of Health 1990; Centers for Disease Control 1990a). And aside from

Table 4.2 Heterosexual Contact Patterns of South Bronx
Women: Characteristics of Current Sex Partners (CSP)
(N = 429)

CSP	Age of woman				
	Less than 20	20-24	25-29	30-34	35 and over
Age: median	21	26	30	34	39
range	15-30	19-55	20-55	23-60	28-56
% of age 25-34:	12%	46%	64%	69%	17%
% of same race/ ethnicity as woman	90%	86%	93%	93%	84%

Zip code of residence of CSP				
Same	Adjacent	South Bronx	Other Bronx	Total Bronx
41%	18%	11%	12%	82%

Source: Drucker et al 1989b.

the consequent high rates of pediatric AIDS within these areas, high HIV prevalence rates among women also implies the potential for further transmission to male sexual partners who may not be drug users. While the efficiency of sexual transmission of HIV is greater from males to females (as is the case with most STDs), some evidence now exists to suggest that the bidirectional transmission seen in Africa and the Caribbean is occurring in NYC (Chiasson et al. 1990; Steigbigel et al. 1987). Some of the risk factors associated with risk of female-to-male transmission—such as concurrent STDs, use of intra-uterine devices or birth-control pills, and lack of circumcision—are now better understood (Kreiss 1990), and the next step in the evolution of the epidemic is most likely to occur in the inner-city areas just described (Drucker 1990).

Diffusion Outward

While the most noticeable initial effect of high levels of HIV infection in the population of urban minority communities may be a sharp rise in the incidence of new infections within these specific neighborhoods, the situation is not static: within several years, there must be some diffusion of infection to adjacent areas. Recent data from the screening of U.S. military applicants illustrates this (Gardner and Brundage 1989). The geographic areas showing the most rapid increase in the rate of HIV infection among recruits are the counties immediately adjacent to those urban areas with the highest absolute prevalence levels of HIV—the suburban counties surrounding NYC, San Francisco, Miami, and Dallas/Fort Worth.

Even within high risk groups, such as IV drug users, this pattern of geographic diffusion can be seen graphically. For example, the rates of HIV infection among methadone patients tested in New Jersey and Connecticut were found to be an inverse function of distance from the NYC epicenter. (See figures 4.4 and 4.5.) This pattern of diffusion is based on the manner in which people buy drugs in the central city areas and then transport them back out to the suburbs and to outlying districts. The travel involved in purchasing drugs may accompany exposure to HIV via needle sharing (to sample wares) or drug-associated sexual contacts in another locale. And, of course, the geographic overlap of drug-using and needle-sharing networks and the small but significant nonexclusivity of race/ethnicity among sexual contacts fosters wider diffusion of any infectious agent. The work of D'Aquila and his colleagues in New Haven (D'Aquila et al. 1987) illustrates this pattern eloquently. The rate of HIV infection among methadone patients tested in several Connecticut cities is an inverse function of auto mileage from NYC. (See figure 4.5.)

Finally, an important additional mechanism for the geographic diffusion of HIV beyond the inner city is associated with migration patterns and the characteristics of social and family networks of African-Americans and Hispanics—many of which bridge geographically distant areas. These social networks create a powerful surrogate of actual proximity and also function to bring populations of some quite distant localities into frequent and intimate association with populations living in AIDS-endemic urban areas. For NYC, the most dramatic instance of this phenomenon can be seen in the Puerto Rican population, which has the highest rates of HIV of any ethnic

Figure 4.4. Rates of HIV Infection among Methadone Patients in New Jersey

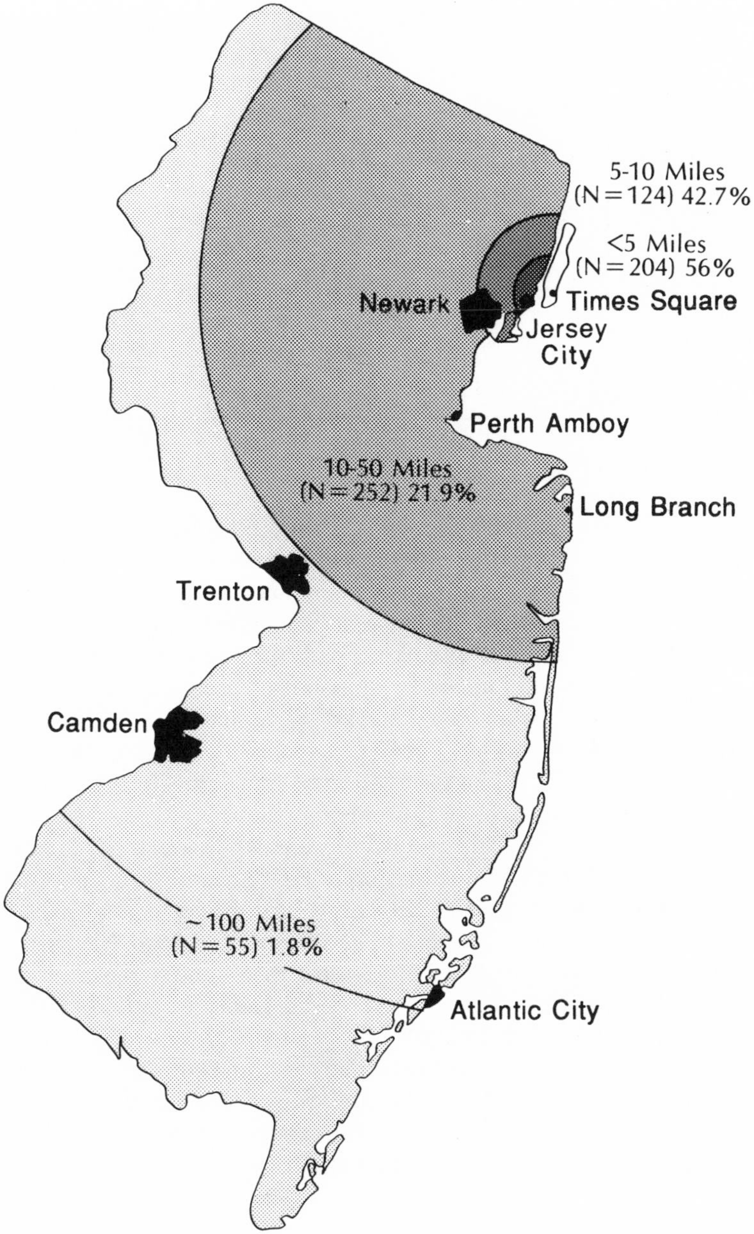

5-10 Miles
(N=124) 42.7%

<5 Miles
(N=204) 56%

Newark

Times Square

Jersey City

Perth Amboy

10-50 Miles
(N=252) 21.9%

Long Branch

Trenton

Camden

~100 Miles
(N=55) 1.8%

Atlantic City

**Figure 4.5. Rates of HIV Infection among Methadone
Patients in Four Connecticut Cities**

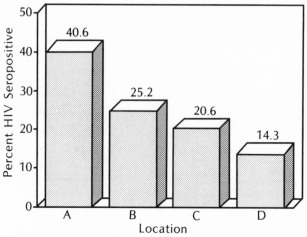

group (Selik et al. 1989; Menendez et al. 1990). This group's close
and ongoing ties with the island of Puerto Rico, through continued residence of many family members of origin and easy and
inexpensive travel via the low-cost "air bridge" (Lambert, *New
York Times,* May 1990), assure a steady stream of travelers. This
pattern may be amplified by the special problems associated
with particular risk factors for HIV—drug use or teenage pregnancy. Drug users often move in response to pressures associated with their addiction, traveling home to Puerto Rico to get
off drugs or to escape legal problems stemming from criminal
activities in NYC. This mobility is a clear mechanism for increasing the risk of transmission of HIV beyond those circum-
scribed local communities with high HIV prevalence levels.

A similar pattern can be seen for the African-American
population of northeastern cities with their family roots in the
southeastern United States (Virginia, Georgia, and the Car-
olinas) and for the African-American population of Chicago
with roots and connections in the Mississippi Delta and the deep
South. In the Atlantic states, migrant farm labor plays an
important role in the spread of the disease. Clusters of AIDS
cases (implying pockets of infection) are already evident in

Georgia and South Carolina (Centers for Disease Control 1990a), and recently these southern cases have been shown to be undercounted or underreported by as much as 50 percent (Lambert 1989d), indicating that the problem is even more advanced than was thought. These examples of the ways in which social patterns of HIV prevalence determine potential geographic diffusion suggest that the current high concentration of HIV infection in the heterosexual minority populations of some American inner-city communities is no assurance of invulnerability for adjacent regions or even for very distant ones.

Impact on Local Health Services

As Peter Gould points out in his chapter, an immediate consequence of the high concentration of AIDS-case incidence in an area is its impact on local hospital and health care services. By the end of 1989, over 2,000 people with AIDS or suspected AIDS occupied hospital beds in NYC each day (Health Systems Agency 1989)—7 percent of the city's total medical/surgical bed capacity of 27,000. This figure is expected to grow to 10-15 percent of that capacity by 1992 (Alderman et al. 1988). On a regular basis, since 1985, approximately 20-25 percent of all those individuals diagnosed and still alive with AIDS in NYC, have been in the hospital on any given day (Drucker et al. 1987). Of course, all the old demands on that system—the needs of the very old and the very young, its traditional users—do not diminish because of a new epidemic. And several significant new burdens other than AIDS care were placed on the system in the 1980s: demands associated with the deinstitutionalization of patients from New York State psychiatric hospitals in the 1970s, high rates of homelessness, and, most recently, the impact of increased drug traffic with its associated violence, more premature infants requiring neonatal intensive care, and longer-stay "boarder babies" (Bigel Institute 1988). All these problems have increased the background demands on the local health care system just as the AIDS epidemic mounts to its highest levels. Acute care hospital beds are the system's most scarce and expensive resource; in January of 1989, over 1,000 patients were "held" in emergency rooms each day awaiting admission to hospital beds (Vladeck 1990). Finally, the severity of illness associated with most AIDS hospitalizations and the increased quality of care required for such patients means that AIDS patients represent more demand than "average" patients and further strain an understaffed system.

As we climb toward an expected annual incidence of 8,000–10,000 new AIDS cases per year in NYC, by 1992 or 1993 we can anticipate that as many as 4,000 of the city's beds nearly one in six will be occupied by AIDS patients (Health Systems Agency 1989). Recent advances in AIDS therapeutics do seem to be lessening the time spent in hospitals by patients at advanced stages of HIV-related illness (Friedland et al. 1991), but these individuals, by living longer, may yet evidence lifetime patterns of hospital utilization equal to those noted prior to intervention. In addition, another 1,000-2,000 beds may be occupied by patients never diagnosed as having CDC-defined AIDS but hospitalized with HIV-related conditions such as pneumonia or tuberculosis (Stoneburner et al. 1988). In the Bronx, between 1982 and 1986, there was a 130 percent increase in pneumonia hospitalizations among adult men (Drucker et al. 1989b). These were apparently HIV-related and accounted for 42 percent more hospital days than AIDS cases themselves during the same period.

Further, one study of AIDS patients in a large private insurance plan in NYC (Eisenhandler 1989) found that patients diagnosed with AIDS utilized significantly more out-patient and hospital services than those without HIV infection *even prior* to their diagnosis. This amount, equal to 20 percent of their utilization *after* diagnosis, was never noted as "AIDS-related" when it occurred since the utilization preceded formal diagnosis with CDC-defined AIDS, but it illustrates the extent of the demand that HIV-related illness places on the health care system before it becomes evident as CDC-defined AIDS per se.

The hospital system of New York is already under intense financial stress associated with the institution of prospective payment plans based on Diagnosis-Related Groups (DRGs). Chronic staffing shortages and large wage increases in several key staff areas, especially nursing will lessen the buying power of health dollars in New York at the same time as its financial resources are reduced and fewer health care workers choose to work in the city's hospitals (Lambert 1989a). Further, these staff shortages are not evenly distributed between voluntary and municipal hospital and the very different communities they serve. New York's municipal hospitals are located in the midst of the AIDS endemic areas and carry the heaviest burden for care of the city's indigent AIDS patients (Health Systems Agency 1989). They also have the largest number of staff vacancies in nursing, medicine, and other skilled categories and the weakest support infrastructure (e.g., social services, counselors, etc.). At Lincoln Medical and Mental Health Center in the South Bronx, ninety-seven beds were out of service because the NYC Health and Hospitals Corporation could not find enough nurses, and a new fully-equipped AIDS unit in the same hospital could not open for two years for the same reason.

Finally, a particularly troubling and unusual aspect of the American AIDS epidemic is a result of the legislated association between drug addiction and criminality. Because of the increased arrest rate and imprisonment of drug users in New York (over 250,000 are arrested each year), large numbers with HIV infection are entering the state prison system. There is already one AIDS death per day within that system. Studies conducted by the New York State Department of Corrections indicate that 20-25 percent of all new inmates are HIV-infected (Greifinger 1990). Among its 50,000 prison inmates, New York State can anticipate 2,000 new cases of AIDS in the coming year, more AIDS cases than some European nations (e.g., Great Britain) have in their general populations. Prison health services are chronically understaffed and have great difficulty in attracting capable individuals, given the traditional place of prison health services on the margins of medicine and public health.

While the impact of the AIDS epidemic in NYC and our inadequacies in meeting its demands are most evident in relation to acute hospital care services, this problem and the scope of our responsibilities enlarge with the promise of early medical intervention and prophylactic treatment of HIV infection prior to the onset of AIDS (Arno et al. 1989; Volberding et al. 1990). Instead of having "just" 10,000 people to treat for full-blown AIDS, NYC now has over 100,000 HIV-infected people eligible for the potential benefits of early intervention with AZT (azidiothymidine), pentamidine, ddI (dideoxyinosine), and the other new drugs that will surely emerge over the next few years. While these drugs may only serve to defer rather than prevent future hospitalization, they unquestionably promise to improve the length and quality of life of those infected with the AIDS virus. Such treatments do, however, require very substantial levels of medical service not currently available to most of the populations who would be most in need of them—inner-city drug users and their families (Bigel Institute 1988). Thus, AIDS invokes a set of new problems closely linked to many old ones: the maldistribution of health care services as a function of social and economic status is a problem already well recognized in the U.S. but one that will not improve until we demonstrate the political will to change health care from a privilege to a right for all citizens.

Conclusion

These data on the local distribution of AIDS show the unevenness of its distribution and the selectivity of its impact on different people and different communities. Often this pattern reflects the historical injustice and inequality with which this country continues to struggle. But "Common Threads", the subtitle of this volume, reflects that AIDS, in reality, is a common problem for all of us. Indeed, the threads that run through this epidemic are deeply woven into the fabric of American society—social and sexual inequity, drug addiction, and racial discrimination and segregation. But there are other threads that bind us together and draw on some of our basic strengths— a belief in fairness, equal treatment under the law, and the right of all citizens to dignity without regard to their race, ethnicity, or economic circumstances. And we are thus left with a paradox. For even if everyone is not equally affected by the AIDS epidemic now, it is still imperative that we all immediately assume a shared responsibility for its resolution. Otherwise, all too soon, we *will* all feel its impact most directly.

Whether the AIDS epidemic is viewed as the inexorable process of geographic diffusion based on slowly spreading circles of infection from regional epicenters (as in Peter Gould's work) or as a natural consequence of the mobility and freedom of association essential to our American way of life, it is clear that "what goes around comes around." Even the most secure and self-satisfied of us can take no comfort from the devastating, almost surgically specific, local impact of the American AIDS epidemic in its early phases. Like all great epidemics, AIDS does not measure time in years but will unfold over decades and perhaps even centuries.

It is virtually impossible to isolate a sexually transmitted disease in a democratic society. Patterns of residential and social interaction, commerce, education, employment, and migration all assure the diffusion of AIDS out of its initial epicenters. The first job of the social scientist is to illuminate these patterns and the processes which facilitate the epidemic's spread—the waves on which the disease rides. But we must also vigorously advocate using this understanding in determining social and health policy and in allocating resources.

Granted, this is an exceptional time in terms of scientific progress, and we have great hope that a "magic bullet" to cure the disease or a vaccine to prevent it will fall into our laps. But those of us who have worked in public health for years do not count on miracles. We must face the reality of this epidemic and its implications for all of our lives and treat it with the deadly seriousness that it clearly deserves. What this requires in practical terms is recognition that a humane and caring response to those already inflicted with the HIV virus and those closest to them (who share the greatest risk) is not only the "right thing" to do for *their* well-being but is also in the best interests of the larger community. The fact that AIDS demands that we all assume responsibility is not simply a moral precept; it is also a biological necessity.

5

Low-Incidence Community Response to AIDS

EDWIN HACKNEY

The problems of people with AIDS who live in large cities with high incidences of AIDS are difficult enough, but people with AIDS and agencies that attempt to provide support services for those with AIDS in low-incidence communities—like Lexington, Kentucky—face unique difficulties.

Lexington, located 75 miles east of Louisville and 80 miles south of Cincinnati in central Kentucky, is a small city with a combined urban-county (Fayette County) population of 225,000. It is a market and medical resource center for all of central and eastern Kentucky. Lexington has six acute care hospitals, including the University of Kentucky Medical Center Hospital, a general, teaching, and research hospital, as well as two psychiatric and two rehabilitative hospitals. Numerous medical practitioners and specialists are based in Lexington, in contrast to rural areas of the state where there are often few physicians. The Bluegrass Area Development District (ADD) comprises seventeen counties with a total population of 570,000 in a radius of fifty miles. This is generally regarded as the health service delivery area for the region; however, it is not unusual for individuals from 300 miles away to come to Lexington for medical care.

The incidence of AIDS in Kentucky has been among the nation's lowest: the annual incidence rate per 100,000 population for cases reported August 1988 through July 1989 in Kentucky was 3.0, compared to a rate of 1.9 for the previous year

(Centers for Disease Control 1989b). Between 1982 and 1984 there were 22 cases of AIDS reported in Kentucky (0.56 rate) and 66 reported in all of 1985-1986 (1.44 rate). Underreporting was always suspected and was dramatically underscored when a Lexington man with AIDS was featured in a picture and cover story in the *Lexington Herald-Leader* (Oct. 12, 1986) and was discovered to be an unreported case. There were 57 cases of AIDS reported in 1987 in Kentucky, 112 cases in 1988, and 129 cases in 1989. A cumulative total of 477 cases—nine were reported in 1990, through October 31. In addition to underreporting, people requiring medical and social service assistance for AIDS or HIV who are diagnosed elsewhere and return home to Kentucky to live are not reported at all, and their numbers are not known.

Cases of AIDS in Lexington/Fayette County are now included in tabulations for the Bluegrass Area Development District, the Kentucky Department of Epidemiology having found that individual county listings were having the adverse effect of producing fear and discrimination in counties reporting only one or two cases. Fayette County had reported a total of five cases in August 1986. The Bluegrass ADD had reported a total of 20 cases by September 1987, a total of 43 by October 1988, and cumulative totals of 52 through August 1989 and 96 through August 1990. In contrast, Louisville and Jefferson County have a cumulative total of 171 reported cases through October 1990 (Cabinet for Human Resources 1989, 1990).

Community Responses to AIDS

By 1984, AIDS had come to Lexington and central Kentucky, and rumors began to circulate in the local gay community about who was ill and who was dying. Outside the gay community there was mostly silence. One exception was the McKee family. David McKee was from rural Kentucky and was a hemophiliac, one of the first in the nation to contract AIDS. Broke and near death, he was facing discharge from the University Hospital. In desperation, his wife, Stella, contacted the local media. As a result of the media attention, David was able to stay in the hospital until he died in October 1984. Since then, Stella McKee has appeared in a PBS television documentary and has spoken widely in conferences and workshops about the inadequacies of help for people with AIDS, especially hemophiliacs and their families (*Lexington Herald-Leader,* Feb. 19, 1988).

In 1985 a local community response to AIDS was formed. An "alternative test site" was established at the Fayette County Health Department, and blood screening was begun in local blood banks. Initially, testing was not anonymous and was therefore generally avoided. Local physicians in particular disseminated much misinformation, and people were told by their doctors "to test, have no sex for three years and then retest" or "take the test three times in three weeks, and have no sex for six weeks before and during testing." One health worker actually told an anxious female blood donor who had tested positive in routine screening to "kiss your ass good-bye."

A local gay group, Gay and Lesbian Services Organization (GLSO), held a highly publicized workshop on AIDS at the University of Kentucky, with an infectious disease specialist and a health department staff member participating. A series of four Safer Sex AIDS Prevention workshops targeting gay men were held, but these workshops reached a total of only eighty people. Gay hotline volunteers were trained to give information about safer sex and AIDS-related referrals for counseling and medical help. In 1985 the local hospice agency, Hospice of the Bluegrass, trained five volunteers from the gay community in the first step of a continuous volunteer effort. This proved to be premature, and it was not until two years later that patients with AIDS were being released routinely to Hospice to be cared for at home. Grants requested from United Way by GLSO to provide AIDS education and prevention in the gay community were not awarded, and the local United Way representative commented that they did not fund "controversial groups." Another gay-organized group from Louisville, the Community Health Trust, raised $6,500 in Lexington in 1985, donating $1,500 to local AIDS-related work and earmarking $5,000 for Glade House, a proposed residence in Louisville for people with AIDS. By late 1985, complaints about the lack of responsiveness of the local public health authorities to what seemed to be an urgent need in the gay community for prevention education led to a series of meetings between health department staff and local gays. Until then, the only funds for prevention activities were raised at "drag" shows and gay community fund-raisers. Little was accomplished until it was announced in February 1986 that federal funding to the state was to be available for AIDS education and prevention among gays and other "high risk groups." It was either not known or not revealed at that time that this money would be spent hiring an "AIDS coordinator" who would primarily do one-on-one HIV testing. Any money that remained could be used in other educational activities. Although it seemed at the time to local gays (and to the AIDS Action Council, a national watchdog group) that this was a misuse of the federal funds, the same thing was occurring all over the country. As of 1990, the Fayette County Health Department had still not targeted any substantial educational efforts to the gay community of Lexington.

Also in 1985, the local Red Cross began receiving materials from national sources, and St. Joseph Hospital began an ambitious staff campaign to mobilize for AIDS work. The Comprehensive Care Center, a local mental health agency, began staff training in its methadone residential and out-patient chemical dependency programs, and AIDS information sessions became a treatment requirement.

In early 1986 an Episcopal group interested in AIDS joined the negotiations with the health department following a national call for action by Episcopal bishops in December 1985. Their involvement considerably broadened the scope and community base. In March 1986 the AIDS Crisis Task Force of Lexington, Inc. was organized. The health department provided an attorney, a post office box, and incorporation, and tax exemption papers were filed. The stated purposes of the group (ACT-Lexington) were to (1) provide education about AIDS to people with AIDS and their families, to persons in "high risk groups," and to the general public; (2) volunteer to assist people with AIDS and provide "buddies," counseling, and other client service through a network of cooperating provider agencies; and (3) provide support for the "worried well" and those infected but not ill.

ACT-Lexington has acquired state funding over four years

and has really only accomplished goal 1 to any great degree. Inexplicably, a large amount of money remains unspent and is restricted to use for provision of AIDS educational and prevention information and materials. All materials must be preapproved by a state review committee and are distributed almost exclusively through the parent agencies of board members. These incude the health department, the Red Cross, Community Mental Health Center, Veteran's Administration Hospital, University of Kentucky Dean of Students Office, University of Kentucky Out-Patient Psychiatry, Gay and Lesbian Services Organization, and Planned Parenthood. The task force effort has failed to grow and has been seen in the community as basically an extended program of the health department and an information clearinghouse for the community. The Red Cross maintains an AIDS information and referral telephone line for ACT, but its efficacy is unknown and coverage is dependent on Red cross staff and one ACT-Lexington volunteer.

In addition to failing to attract volunteer participation, the ACT board has notably been unable to attract members from the black community. Health department outreach has included more blacks in target audiences, but the importance of volunteerism from the black community has not yet been understood by this board. A sixteen-member advisory board was organized and then neglected and no longer exists in a formal sense. ACT education efforts have been principally those of the staff of the Fayette County Health Department AIDS Team. Efforts were made to involve a truly community-wide sample, and grassroots involvement was encouraged but never materialized. Education efforts of the health department staff have targeted a general public audience but not specific groups. ACT has co-sponsored an AIDS training conference with St. Joseph Hospital, training for nursing home administrators (which unsuccessfully attempted to encourage admissions for people with HIV infection—none of the fifty-three nursing homes in the Bluegrass ADD accept HIV-infected persons), and recently a conference on AIDS for health care professionals working with the mentally retarded and chronically mentally ill. Also, placards have been placed on buses and posters and brochures have been distributed under the auspices of ACT.

In October 1986 a support group was formed for men who were HIV-positive and anxious about AIDS. Having done very little planning, they attempted without success, to meet at the health department and later the mental health center. Participants were fearful of such public places and of being identified and reported. Anonymous testing was new, and distrust was high. The presence of the health department AIDS coordinator who was responsible for much of the HIV counseling proved to be unwise: he was often seen as an extension of the state AIDS reporting apparatus, and because he knew many people in the gay community, people feared being recognized. (Many local gays chose testing in other cities for this reason. This pattern has been noted also in most rural areas where true anonymity is not possible because "everyone knows everyone else.") After a break in the summer of 1987, the support group resumed and has continued meeting weekly at an undisclosed location. Screening is provided by a volunteer social worker, and the group follows a self-help format. A volunteer Buddy Program was formed, co-sponsored by ACT and Hospice. At the first ACT Buddy Training on August 2-3, 1986, fourteen people were trained in patient care, infection control, death and dying, psychosocial issues, and crisis intervention. Follow-up training was held on a monthly basis, but by the end of 1986 only one buddy referral had been made. The program suffered attrition of volunteers through 1987, with only one additional patient referral made that year. Most client contact was by phone, and the referral system remained disorganized.

By mid-1987, the ACT board had shrunk to six members, there was no active fund-raising, volunteers were becoming discouraged because there were few referrals, the ACT Education Committee met irregularly and had no active agenda, interagency competition for available resources caused occasional strain, and the support group was suspended. But perhaps the biggest setback was the "ACT-SMART" campaign in February 1987. The new ACT president, a gay man with AIDS-volunteer experience from another city, had initiated, with health department assistance, a long-awaited AIDS awareness campaign for the local gay community. The campaign featured a small card with safe sex messages, an attached condom, and a proposal to do "home party" safe sex seminars for gay men. The president notified the press of a condom giveaway planned for a local gay bar on Valentine's Day. Not only did the newspaper run a detailed article on the campaign, a television crew showed up the night of the kickoff celebration and brought lights and cameras rolling into the local gay bar. It was an unmitigated disaster. The owner ejected the TV crew and the ACT-SMART table, and many customers fled the scene immediately. The president gave an interview on the sidewalk, explaining on the air that local gays "hadn't learned yet," that many "didn't care," and further that he wanted to have parties in people's homes to teach "creative" ways to "still enjoy safe sex" (Lexington Herald-Leader, Feb. 14, 1987). One could easily get the impression from the ACT president's remarks that local gays were rejecting safe sex and AIDS-prevention efforts. He never regained his credibility, and any attempt to promote programs in the gay community would no longer involve ACT-Lexington. This mistake was an honest one: an openly gay man from a larger urban area was unaccustomed to the attitudes toward homosexuality that exist in more rural areas. He never considered that there might be something wrong with publicly promoting homosexual activity in a state with sodomy laws and blatantly using state-funded materials and condoms to do so. He also disregarded the concern of local closeted gays for whom a television appearance would do great personal harm.

Throughout 1986 and 1987, community activity revolved around training, building community awareness about AIDS, and setting policies for future problems. Most hospitals initiated some kind of training for staff, and numerous articles about AIDS with a focus on local issues appeared in the local press. Calls for "routine" testing of "high-risk groups" and blood transfusion recipients and the discussion of quarantine created controversy (Lexington Herald-Leader, July 30, 1987, and June 2, 1987). The health department and the Fayette County Medical Society distributed brochures to all local physicians detailing recommended counseling for HIV testing, AIDS treatments, and referral resources. The Lexington Clinic and St. Joseph Hospital became primary treatment centers. For the most part, cooperation in resource development and in working with community groups and families to provide a support network for people with HIV disease has been excellent, but at some places, including the University Hospital and out-patient clinics, the response has been quite different. Referral to community support networks has been resisted, patients referred to clinics have at times been turned away if they could not pay a fee, and the insistence that university-affiliated medical facilities are not for indigent care has often placed a serious barrier to treatment for poor and uninsured patients. When a federally funded Clinical Trials Unit opened at the University of Cincinnati, many patients were referred there. The reluctance of the local university medical center to develop programs for people with AIDS is only just beginning to improve. Both the Veteran's Administration Hospital and University of Kentucky Psychiatry have had "HIV teams" in place for some time, and in 1989 a task force was formed to include various departments of the medical school and hospital complex to begin to coordinate work with people with AIDS. Whether planning will include the community outside or not remains to be seen; clearly, much needs to be done to help Lexington's largest medical complex respond to the community around it.

In February 1987 the Fayette County School Board passed an AIDS policy and approved programming for teaching AIDS in the schools, with, however, restrictions on the discussion of birth control and homosexuality. Teams of second-year medical students from the University of Kentucky Medical School found that Fayette County is the only county—out of the more than twenty counties where they instruct eighth graders—that required their curriculum to be altered. In this innovative program, medical and pharmacy students have generally had a good response to their efforts at AIDS education in the schools.

Jail AIDS policies in Lexington have gradually begun to evolve, but HIV-infected prisoners have been subjected to harassment and discrimination. Furthermore, prisoners have been released because they have HIV-infection, and some area jails have refused to accept HIV-positive prisoners. There have been no serious difficulties with funeral homes and burial policies, although families often have closed funerals to prevent acknowledging AIDS or facing curiosity.

A branch of the East Central AIDS Education and Training Center (ECAETC) was formed in 1987 with the University of Kentucky Department of Allied Health and has become an excellent resource for health and social service professionals throughout the state. And in 1986 Nazareth Home in Louisville was approved to accept AIDS referrals, with two beds reserved for that purpose. It remains the only nursing home in Kentucky and one of the few in the nation that accepts AIDS referrals (Louisville *Courier-Journal,* July 9, 1986). Glade House, a residence for people with AIDS in Louisville, opened in 1986 and soon accepted its first referral from Lexington.

Outreach to blacks became a priority in 1987, and the AIDS Task Force asked Professor Ivan Banks of the University of Kentucky to consult. The health department announced it was exploring ways to reach the black community (*Lexington Herald-Leader,* July 20, 1987)—a representative from the National AIDS Network came to speak, and a small, family-oriented social services program in the black community (Family Learning and Development) received some AIDS education funding—but there has been very little activity.

The community mental health center has had eight clinicians trained in pre- and post-test HIV counseling and has worked out an arrangement with the health department to refer clients who request anonymous testing. Regular risk-reduction sessions for clients are held in all the residential and out-patient programs serving IV drug users, and there has been a cautious response from this population. Although it is in the early stages, AIDS transmission among IV drug users and their sexual partners is now a fact in central Kentucky.

Two further education efforts occurred in the latter half of 1987. An attempt was made to organize a community education forum and galvanize public opinion through inviting a nationally-known speaker such as Surgeon General C. Everett Koop and through telephone calls and other types of contacts to local community leaders, charity organizers, and socialites. Lexington and the Bluegrass have always benefited from highly visible and generous philanthropy from the local gentry, and "old money" is a prominent feature of the central Kentucky social structure. The organizing effort, begun as a project with the University of Kentucky College of Social Work, was largely unsuccessful in tapping the upper echelon of the social strata, and it was clearly demonstrated that AIDS was not an acceptable charity yet in this locality, nor was it really even considered a subject to be discussed in polite company. Eventually a committee evolved composed of a member of the local medical society auxiliary, a Community Action-Lexington, Fayette County (CALF) staffer, an Episcopal church member, a teacher, a dentist, a Catholic priest, a sociology professor, and the social worker who directed the project. An honorary chairperson had previous community board experience and was a member of the local horse farm society. The group met several times, endorsed a community AIDS Education Forum plan, and extended an invitation to Surgeon General Koop. After his office declined the invitation, the group seemingly lost interest and did not pursue any further goals. University of Kentucky social workers David Royse and S. Dhooper have conducted two studies showing widespread fear of AIDS among professionals and students at the University of Kentucky (Royse et al. 1987) and among a statewide population surveyed in 1987 (Dhooper and Royse 1989). Particularly important was the misinformation about how AIDS could be spread. The Bluegrass State Poll (Louisville *Courier-Journal,* Nov. 6, 1988) found that Kentuckians' AIDS knowledge had increased, partly because of the June 1988 federal government mailing of the brochure "Understanding AIDS."

In August 1987 a representative from AIDS Volunteers of Cincinnati was invited to Lexington for a presentation of the "Stop AIDS" safe sex workshop, a San Francisco-based program active in Cincinnati. A wide cross-section of the gay community was invited, and a restatement of the goal of providing risk reduction and AIDS education in the gay community became a theme. Out of this "stop AIDS" meeting evolved the AIDS Volunteers of Lexington (AVOL), patterned closely after the Cincinnati model.

AVOL organizational meetings began in September 1987, and officers and a board of directors were elected. Stated goals were simple and open-ended: "to provide education to the Lexington community on the AIDS epidemic as well as safer sex

techniques," "to provide a support system for people with
AIDS," and "to provide whatever services that its membership
believes is necessary to help the Lexington Community deal
with the AIDS crisis" (AVOL 1987). As a grass-roots organization, AVOL began with a strong emphasis on the needs of
"consumers"—people with AIDS or HIV disease—and their
input was actively sought. The board decided to allow the Lexington Gay and Lesbian Services Organization to assume fiscal
and corporate control in order to take advantage of GLSO's tax-
exempt status and experience in handling funds. A federally-
funded HERR grant was applied for, and an education program
targeting local gay bars was begun. The Buddy Program was
reorganized and reactivated with new volunteers. The HIV support group (and other client-direct service activities from ACT)
was brought under the AVOL umbrella, and materials such as
self-care manuals, AIDS newsletters, and up-to-date health referral information were provided to participants and members.
The goal was to have access to the same level of information
available in New York or San Francisco. Although there is still
great fear and many choose not to associate with the group, the
effort has been very successful. In 1988 the group accepted
participation by a person with AIDS, and now the group is
composed of people with AIDS, ARC, and HIV. AVOL Buddies
continued to be trained in the Hospice training program and are
thus automatically certified to work with Hospice if their referrals become Hospice-eligible.

During 1988 an increase in family requests for support
resulted in an AVOL-sponsored family support group that has
continued to meet weekly and is facilitated by a social work
professor. This group also only became viable when prospective
participants were reassured that group meeting locations would
not be revealed publicly. By early 1989, because of increased
requests for services for women, a support group for women, the
Women's AIDS Project, was organized and co-sponsored by the
University of Kentucky College of Nursing. This has begun as a
more or less autonomous program and has yet to realize a great
number of referrals, encountering the same hesitancy other
programs have faced.

Also during 1988, lack of housing for people with AIDS

began to be recognized as a problem when three requests for housing were received. The AVOL board decided to seek housing for two residents and a manager following the Glade House model in Louisville. The program, named Solomon House, opened in January 1989 and soon received a $5,000 grant from the Lexington-Fayette Urban County Government.

As of the end of 1989, Solomon House had had only one resident for three months, and decisions had to be made as to whether to keep this costly project open (1989 projected budget was $15,000) or to adopt a less costly "scattered site" model for housing. It was not anticipated that so many families and other resources would be available locally to house people with AIDS. Furthermore, Louisville has absorbed some of the demand from Lexington. However, with increased demands for housing, Solomon House has remained open and fully utilized through autumn 1990.

Unlike the AIDS Task Force, AVOL has made fund-raising and volunteer recruitment a major priority. There have been several successful community-wide campaigns: raffles, dances, cocktail parties, and yard sales. A current project involves using volunteer labor to paint and repair a house under a government-funded neighborhood improvement program and donating the payment to AVOL. With these funds, AVOL has been able to provide limited financial assistance in emergencies to people with AIDS and their families. It was anticipated that the need for funds for medication would be a much greater expense with the September 1989 expiration of federally-funded AZT assistance and no state funding available as an alternative. It is a deplorable commentary on the present health care system that we must have yard sales to provide money for prescriptions and medical care for people with AIDS. A medication assistance program was refunded, however, and it includes an expanded list of drugs for persons in need. AVOL also continues to provide financial assistance for medication.

In recent months, many positive changes have occurred in Lexington's fight against AIDS. AVOL has incorporated as an independent entity, a Women's AIDS Project has been initiated with the University of Kentucky College of Nursing, and there has been continued discussion about outreach to women, the black community, and IV drug users. A minority outreach worker has been hired by the health department and will be working with Professor Banks and the Family Learning and Development Center to help develop programs in the black community. In March 1989 the Federal Office of Civil Rights challenged the Cabinet for Human Resources to revise its regulations so that persons with communicable diseases are not subject to discrimination in admission to long-term care facilities. A thorough set of recommendations covering this and several other AIDS-related issues has been proposed in a report by the HIV Human Services Working Group for the Cabinet for Human Resources and its successor, a volunteer advisory group called the Statewide HIV Planning Action Council. A CHR plan for regional care coordinators who provide case management and resource development for people with HIV disease was funded by the 1990 legislature and should further expand the range of services, especially in rural areas.

The University of Kentucky has embarked on an ambitious AIDS awareness campaign with students and staff. One of its more controversial features was the placing of condoms in vending machines in dormitories, but this has apparently met with resistance, and many students report they are not willing to use the machines for fear of embarrassment. Transylvania University has had a much more low-profile AIDS prevention campaign.

Summarizing with Statistics

Since 1986, there has been a generally steady increase in AIDS direct service requests in Lexington, tables 5.1-5.3 indicate. (The figures in tables 5.1-5.3 are based upon the records of ACT-Lexington prior to October 1987 and of AVOL support services since that date.) The 138 referrals represent the contacts made within Kentucky (table 5.1). Of this total, about 60 percent (80) came from Fayette County, 15 percent (21) came from contiguous counties, and the remainder (31 referrals, or 22 percent) came from rural counties in eastern and central Kentucky. Another 25 referrals originated in other states (some of whom were returning to Kentucky), including eight from California.

Table 5.1 AIDS-Related Referrals in Lexington by Status, 1986-1989

Year	HIV +	ARC/AIDS	Family support	Total referrals
1986	8	6	1	15
1987	12	9	6	27
1988	11	13	9	33
1989	18	26	19	63
Total	49	54	35	138

Sources: ACT-Lexington and AVOL.

Table 5.2 Support Group Referrals in Lexington, 1986-1989

Year	HIV +	ARC/AIDS	Total referrals
1986	6	0	6
1987	6	3	9
1988	6	5	11
1989	10	12	22
Total	28	20	48

Sources: ACT-Lexington and AVOL.

Table 5.3 Buddy Program Referrals in Lexington, 1985-1989

Year	Accepted referrals	Patient-declined referrals	Number of volunteers
1985	0	0	5
1986	1	0	14
1987	1	0	6
1988	3	6	5
1989	12	7	9
Total	17	13	39

Sources: ACT-Lexington and AVOL.

Nearly 65 percent (89 of 138) of the total referrals through September 1989 have been white males (table 5.1). Only seven of the total referrals (5 percent) were black. Among the HIV-positive group, three were females (one of whom was black) and four were black males. Among the ARC/AIDS group, seven referrals were female, two of whom were black. Females comprised the majority of those who sought family support: 29 in this group were white females and six were white males.

Support group referrals have increased slightly since 1986, from six in that year to more than triple that during 1989 (table 5.2). Of those referrals participating in the support group, one-fourth (12 of 48) commute from another county. Five deaths have occurred during 1989 among those participating in this group.

The number of accepted referrals in the AVOL Buddy Program has also increased since its inception in 1985, but a number of patients have declined referrals (table 5.3) for a number of reasons, the most prevalent reason being homophobia. Patients and their families often perceive any AIDS-related service as gay-oriented and therefore undesirable. The number of volunteers for this program is of course related to the number of accepted referrals, and in no case has a request for a volunteer been refused. Volunteer training is coordinated twice a year with Hospice of the Bluegrass, and follow-up volunteer training and support takes place on a monthly basis.

Conclusions, Recommendations, and Considerations

Finally, there are several general points to be made about AIDS education and service delivery in Lexington and central Kentucky:

(1) Rural low-incidence AIDS service models differ significantly from those in urban high-incidence areas. Lexington has been described as a "big town run by small town people." Groups function as friendship or "good-old-boy" networks. As noted by Rounds (1988), such groups consider religion, traditional values, and conformity important and are less tolerant of diversity. "Taking care of your own" is a cherished value, and entire families often stay in hospitals with the patient. This can lead to some strained living conditions but has provided shelter for

family members when nothing else was available. There has been an absence of active government involvement by elected officials at any level, and the lack of political support for AIDS has translated into a lack of leadership. There is, in fact, active organized political opposition to the use of public funds to assist persons with AIDS. One Kentucky legislator, having commented that he didn't see what the fuss was about, declared that Kentucky had "more cases of measles than AIDS" (Mason 1989).

(2) There has been a great ambivalence among professionals working with AIDS. There is a lack of support for helpers, who face high risk for burnout, stress, ostracism, and discrimination. Also, persistent reports are received by AVOL of persons denied dental, medical, or legal services by professionals who fear infection. With mandated education for health professionals provided in 1990 legislation, it is hoped that this situation will improve. The same legislation, HB425, the "Mason Bill," provides for relief from discrimination in housing, employment, and public accomodations.

(3) The urban gay "out of the closet" mentality conflicts with a more rural "be discreet" or "survival" model. Invisibility has always been the price gays must pay for tolerance in Kentucky, and AIDS upsets this balance, provoking homophobia and forcing upon the public an uncomfortable awareness of their gay neighbors. The homophobia of the region is perhaps most poignantly demonstrated by "Smear the Queer," a popular Lexington children's playground game also known as "dodge ball." There is also a local history of religious bigotry and religious conflict generally, as a quick glance at the local letters to the editor demonstrates. It would be a serious oversight to omit bigotry as a characteristic of rural areas like central Kentucky, and much hatred and fear must be recognized as a major barrier to developing AIDS services locally. Internalized fears and homophobic self-hatred in gay persons with AIDS are often fueled by disapproving families, and the volunteer helper is often faced with the dilemma of trying to help people live who prefer to hide and die. One wonders if shame can also kill. A concentrated and aggressive anti-prejudice campaign would most likely benefit the area.

(4) Rounds (1988) has pointed out the problems of rural

AIDS organizations being seen as gay organizations, posing credibility problems with referral and funding sources. Some of the strongest criticism that the local AIDS services groups are "too gay" seems to be coming from professionals who are gay themselves. Over 70 percent of the cases of AIDS in Kentucky have been gay men,and the rate has been steady. There have also been criticisms from other professionals that gays are not "trustworthy" or competent to handle referrals of non-gays and that gay men (or any men) are not appropriate to handle referrals of women. Nonprofessional volunteers are seen as not having enough skill to deal with AIDS-related issues.

(5) The strong local focus on "long hospital stays and certain death" has shifted to a focus on "shorter stays and Hospice home care and certain death." Health professionals have shown great reluctance to promote survival as an option for people with AIDS. Many people testing in medical facilities are given the death pronouncement for the positive HIV test alone. Support for people with AIDS has become a national movement, and promoting hope for survival is a key component to any AIDS support program. One not so subtle reaction among health professionals and even families has been to agree "how much better off he'd be dead" when the patient is not even seriousy sick yet. It remains uncertain just how deep the willingness to care for people with AIDS goes, and any undercurrent of resistance by helpers can result in great despair and frustration for people struggling with AIDS.

(6) Kentucky's AIDS crisis has been complicated by two preexisting crises: the crisis in long-term and home care for the elderly and the crisis in rural care of all kinds. One recent study says that 20 percent of AIDS cases are rural (Joint Task Force 1989). Kentucky has a doctor shortage in the rural counties and too many doctors in urban areas. A long and controversial state freeze on nursing home expansion has made long-term care problematic even *without* AIDS. In many areas of the state, rural medical care is inconvenient or nonexistent and home care is not an option.

(7) Present research needs include a thorough study of government agency and grass-roots activity in AIDS education and service delivery and a comprehensive needs assessment to de-

termine local needs and to identify gaps in services. With the urgent need for funding for medication and the limited Medicaid eligibility of persons needing AZT and other medications early in their infection, a research study is needed to compare local hospital costs for AIDS treatment with out-patient medication treatment costs for healthy HIV-positive persons. Home health and Hospice costs should also be computed. Hypothetically, this information could present a case for legislative action to fund early treatment costs and thereby prevent more expensive in-patient care with progressive illness.

(8) On November 1, 1989, "HIV disease" reporting by physicians began using coded data under new Cabinet for Human Resources regulations. This change has not been publicly discussed, and a clear public airing of the issues involved in this change, particularly the effect on confidentiality, is needed.

(9) Epidemiologists studying AIDS must consider the "human impact" of their findings and predictions. It is important that information like the forecast of ultimate fatality for all persons with AIDS be carefully assessed for its effect on people living with AIDS. Such predictions rob people of hope, create despair, and make survival more difficult for those whose struggle is already difficult enough.

(10) Finally, in rural areas, the identification by location (county, town) of cases of AIDS for epidemiological purposes must be assessed in terms of the impact on the locality. In one Kentucky county reporting a case of AIDS, a local resident was the subject of gossip and harassment until declaring in the media that she did not have AIDS. Much remains to be understood about the social impact of AIDS epidemiologic information, and a balance is needed among facts, dismal predictions, and hope.

6

AIDS: Socioepidemiologic Responses to an Epidemic

WILLIAM W. DARROW

Principles and methods of sociology and epidemiology have been applied to our understanding of the epidemic of Acquired Immunodeficiency Syndrome (AIDS) since the outbreak was first recognized in 1981. This chapter presents a series of successive socioepidemiologic investigations that were conducted before the identification of Human Immunodeficiency Virus (HIV) as the etiologic agent of AIDS in 1984: a case study, a case-control study, and a cluster investigation of homosexual and bisexual men with AIDS who were linked by sexual contact. Later in the chapter, more recent studies of the heterosexual transmission of HIV and behavior change will be described and some suggestions for future research will be offered.

Sociology has been defined as the systematic study of interpersonal behavior (Merton 1965). The smallest unit of analysis in sociology is the dyad: a couple involved in interaction. Sexual relationships are well-suited for sociologic analysis because they usually involve two people interacting with one another in socially patterned ways (Gagnon and Simon 1973).

Epidemiology has been defined as the systematic study of the incidence, distribution, and control of diseases in human populations (MacMahon and Pugh 1970). Most epidemiologists have been trained in medicine and have strong backgrounds in research methods and statistics. Epidemiologists resemble sociologists in that both study groups of people and examine patterns, but epidemiologists tend to look at the physical or demographic characteristics of individuals and argue for the "biological plausibility" of observed relationships.

Epidemiologic models examine relationships between three major variables: the biologic characteristics of human hosts, the agents that cause disease, and the physical environment (Coe 1970). By understanding the properties of these variables and the linkages between them, epidemiologists hope to control or eradicate the diseases they study through the application of clinical, preventive, and environmental medicine. In contrast, most sociologists are reluctant to interfere with social processes and to impose social controls on populations chosen for study (Cohen 1966).

A model for the sociologic study of sexually transmitted diseases (STDs) might include four major variables: health consumers who become infected and seek or require medical services, health providers who offer medical care, social exchanges among and between those who acquire or treat diseases, and the sociocultural environments in which those exchanges occur (Darrow 1976). Obviously, there are similarities between the epidemiologic and sociologic models in that both are interested in the behaviors of human beings and both carefully consider environmental conditions. Epidemiologists, however, tend to emphasize biologic and chemical factors, while sociologists tend to ignore the effects of biologic or chemical agents and often include the behavioral patterns of medical practitioners as well as "hosts" and "susceptibles" in their paradigms (Freidson 1976).

Social epidemiology combines elements of sociology and epidemiology to assess how interpersonal behavior influences the incidence, distribution, and control of diseases (such as AIDS) in human populations; thus, social epidemiologists try to answer questions about how diseases enter into human populations and then are recognized as such. They also study how diseases are spread or are inhibited from spreading in human populations (Darrow, Gorman, and Glick 1986).

Fortunately, some support is now emerging for research on the social epidemiology of HIV disease. Almost half of the Public Health Service's budget of $1.3 billion for fiscal year 1989 supported biomedical research at the National Institutes of Health

Figure 6.1. Centers of Disease Control:
FY 1989 HIV Prevention Activities

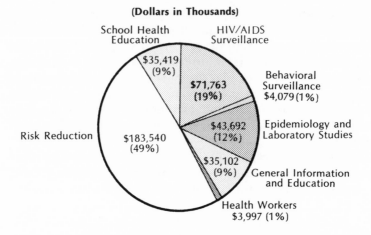

(Dollars in Thousands)

School Health
Education

HIV/AIDS
Surveillance

$35,419
(9%)

$71,763
(19%)

Behavioral
Surveillance
$4,079 (1%)

$43,692
(12%)

Epidemiology and
Laboratory Studies

Risk Reduction

$183,540
(49%)

$35,102
(9%)

General Information
and Education

Health Workers
$3,997 (1%)

Figure 6.2. Spectrum of HIV Disease

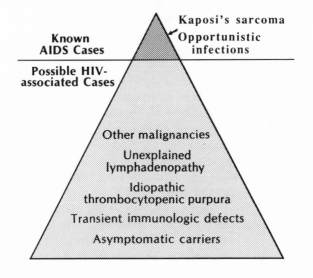

Known
AIDS Cases

Kaposi's sarcoma
Opportunistic
infections

Possible HIV-
associated Cases

Other malignancies

Unexplained
lymphadenopathy

Idiopathic
thrombocytopenic purpura

Transient immunologic defects

Asymptomatic carriers

(NIH), but some of the funding at NIH and elsewhere was used to study the socioepidemiologic aspects of AIDS (Centers for Disease Control 1989a).

The budget for the Centers for Disease Control (CDC) has grown in the past decade from $288 million in fiscal year 1981 to a projected $1 billion in fiscal year 1990, in large part because of funding increases for HIV surveillance, research, and prevention programs. Currently, almost half of CDC's HIV prevention budget (49 percent) supports risk-reduction activities, such as counseling and HIV-antibody testing through state and local health departments; $43 million (12 percent) is used to support epidemiologic and laboratory studies, and another $4 million (1 percent) is used to support "behavioral surveillance activities," primarily the "AIDS Knowledge and Attitudes" supplement to the *Health Interview Survey* conducted by the National Center for Health Statistics (see figure 6.1).

AIDS activities at CDC are restricted to surveillance, epidemiologic and laboratory studies, and prevention services. Included in the HIV/AIDS prevention services are general information and education, risk-reduction activities, and programs aimed at school- and college-age youth. Although the 1989 budget allows expenditures for "behavioral surveillance" and "behavioral epidemiology," there is no line item for social or behavioral research. Therefore, sociologic research at CDC must be closely tied to the "social epidemiology" of HIV disease.

Socioepidemiologic Research on AIDS

In April 1981, CDC began to receive reports of a highly unusual and apparently acquired immune disorder that was primarily striking previously healthy, relatively young homosexual men in major metropolitan areas of the United States (Curran et al. 1982). The CDC Task Force on AIDS was formed to investigate the outbreak, and specialists in infectious diseases, molecular virology, environmental medicine, parasitology, immunology, and sociology (among others) were asked to join. The major objective of the task force was to find the cause of AIDS.

Scientists developed a number of hypotheses to explain the origin of AIDS. One possibility was that the disorder was caused by a new or previously unrecognized infectious agent, but other possibilities such as immunologic overload from repeated infections or exposure to a toxic substance had to be considered. The relationship between "agent X," the unknown cause of AIDS, and the clinical manifestations of its effects on the human immune system had to be explored systematically. Studies were designed in sequence to solve some of the mysteries of AIDS. First, patients had to be carefully characterized before an acceptable, working case definition of AIDS could be established; then, cases and carefully matched controls had to be compared for clues as to the essential differences between the two groups. Finally, additional investigations had to be conducted to validate or refute initial findings.

After examining, interviewing, and collecting specimens from thirty-one people with AIDS in the summer of 1981, researchers formulated a "working" case definition of AIDS (Centers for Disease Control 1982). This definition would change several times as further evidence was gathered, but there was initial agreement to conduct surveillance for additional cases based on three criteria: (1) existence of biopsy-proven Kaposi's sarcoma and/or biopsy– or culture-proven life-threatening opportunistic infection; (2) disease manifestation in previously healthy persons less than sixty years of age; and (3) exclusion of patients with conditions known to cause immunosuppression, such as congenital immunodeficiency, lymphoreticular malignancy, and therapy with immunosuppressive agents.

Although the research community generally accepted the working case definition, many investigators realized that recognized AIDS cases could represent just the tip of an iceberg (Drotman and Curran 1984). Other conditions being seen at that time could also be caused by the same etiologic agent and could represent additional manifestations of its deleterious effects (see figure 6.2). Furthermore, scientists postulated an asymptomatic state of infection, and some believed that the agent could be transmitted by infected persons who had no signs or symptoms of disease.

The task force conducted a case-control study in late 1981 comparing epidemiologic and laboratory findings for 50 homosexual men with Kaposi's sarcoma or *Pneumocystis carinii* pneumonia with 120 homosexual men with no evidence of AIDS. Research participants were matched for race and age group and drawn from STD clinics or private physician practices in the same four cities where the cases had been diagnosed (Jaffe et al. 1983). Factor analysis suggested that the major differences between men with AIDS and men with no evidence of AIDS were with respect to the numbers of recent sex partners and recent episodes of STDs. The evidence for common environmental exposures or other possibilities was less compelling.

After one of the research subjects in the case-control study died in March 1982, his former roommate and lover called a medical officer assigned to the Los Angeles Department of Public Health and told him the following story.

In October 1979, a gay and lesbian services organization held its annual fund-raising banquet in Los Angeles. Over eight hundred people attended. Tickets sold for $150 per person, or $1,500 for a table of ten. One benefactor bought ten tickets and gave them to five couples, none of whom had previously met the other couples. As illustrated in figure 6.3, *A* sat with his companion of three years, *B; C* sat with his companion of three years, *D; E* sat with his companion of 21 years, *F;* and the other couples (not designated by letters) later joined them at the same table.

In the summer of 1980, *E* and *F* decided to have a small party by their backyard pool. They invited *C, D,* and a third person, later described as "a $50 trick off Santa Monica Boulevard," to join them (figure 6.4). During the course of the evening, each man present had sexual contacts with the others who were there.

In October 1980, two of the men who had met one year earlier at the banquet began to feel ill (figure 6.5). *B* and *F* felt weak and tired and inexplicably began to lose weight. Subsequently, *B* and *F* developed *Pneumocystis carinii* pneumonia and died. *B* died on October 6, 1981, and *F* died on February 6, 1982. *D* developed lymphadenopathy in July of 1981, was diagnosed as having Kaposi's sarcoma in August, and died on March 6, 1982. When *D* died on the same day of the month as *B* and *F, C* put the dates together ("666"), thought it was an ominous sign, and called a member of the CDC Task Force on AIDS to tell him

Figure 6.3.	Figure 6.4.
Homosexual Couples at a Los Angeles Fund-Raising Banquet, October 1979	**Sexual Contacts of Two Homosexual Couples and a Male Prostitute, Summer 1980**

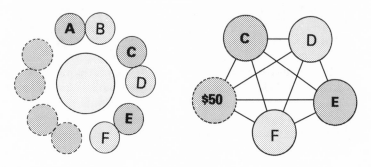

Figure 6.5.

Sickness and Death of Three Individuals Who Met at Los Angeles Fund-Raising Banquet in 1979

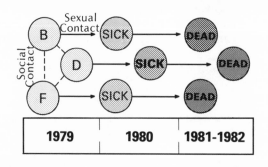

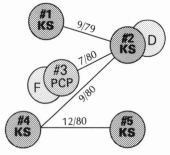

Figure 6.6.

Dates of Sexual Contacts of Some of the First AIDS Cases in Los Angeles

Figure 6.7.

Out-of-California Case Linked by Sexual Contact to Three Early Cases in Los Angeles

Figure 6.8.

Out-of-California Case Linked to Other Early Cases in Los Angeles

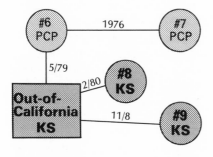

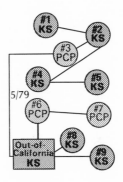

Figure 6.9.

Out-of-California Case Directly Linked to Four of the First Twelve Known Los Angeles Cases and Four of Twenty Known Cases in New York City

Figure 6.10.

Forty of 248 Homosexual Men Reported to CDC as Having AIDS Linked by Sexual Exposure, April 1982

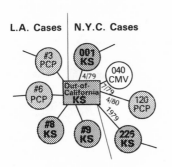

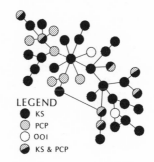

this story. It is important to note that since *B* was not at the pool party and *C* and *E* appeared to be well, a common environmental exposure (e.g., the air at the banquet or a contaminant in the pool water) was ruled out as the cause of the diseases.

Of the nineteen cases of AIDS reported in Los Angeles among homosexual men (as of April 1982), my colleague in Los Angeles and I were able to gather some information on sixteen and sexual contact information on thirteen. Nine of the thirteen could be linked by one or more sexual exposures within five years of the onset of symptoms to at least one other reported case. In figure 6.6, *D* appears as Patient #2, *F* as Patient #3, and the date of their sexual exposure is indicated: July 1980. When we interviewed *C, E,* and other persons with AIDS (or their close companions) in Los Angeles, we discovered that Patient #2 had also had sexual relations with Patient #1 in September 1979 and with Patient #4 in September 1980.

Patients #6 and #7 were lovers in 1976 before they moved to Los Angeles and shared certain sex partners after they arrived. Patients #8 and #9 had never met when we interviewed them on April 7, 1982. We were very surprised when each one told us that he had had sexual contact with the same out-of-California case; Patient #8 had had contact in February and Patient #9 in November 1980 (figure 6.7). We were astounded when, on the same day, the companion of a third case in Los Angeles said that his roommate had had sexual contacts with two friends of this same out-of-California case.

After we learned about the importance of the out-of-California case, I made arrangements to interview him. When I spoke with him over the telephone, he told me that he had had sexual contacts with two additional cases in Los Angeles: Patient #6 and someone we had interviewed earlier, Patient #3 (figure 6.8). Thus, it was through the candor of the out-of-California case that we were able to link together nine cases of AIDS in southern California.

When I interviewed the out-of-California case in person, he told me that he had had 250 different sex partners from December 1978 until he developed lymphadenopathy in December 1979, 250 while he felt ill in 1980, and 250 more in 1981. Of these 750 men, he identified 72 (or about 10 percent) by name. More of these (37.5 percent) lived in San Francisco than other cities, but none of his contacts in San Francisco had been reported to CDC as cases. However, four out of twelve in Los Angeles and four out of twenty in New York City were known cases of Kaposi's sarcoma, *Pneumocystis carinii* pneumonia, or other opportunistic infections (figure 6.9).

The earliest exposure dates were given for two cases in New York City, Patient 001 and Patient 226. Both of these men were subsequently connected to other cases. The other two cases from New York City, Patients 040 and 120, had died by the time I tried to reach them.

Of the 248 homosexual men reported to CDC as having AIDS as of April 12, 1982, we were able to link 40 by sexual exposures (Auerbach et al. 1984) (figure 6.10). Evidence gathered during the cluster investigation confirmed findings from the case-control study and strongly suggested that AIDS was caused by a sexually-transmitted pathogen. In 1983, researchers at the Pasteur Institute in Paris and at NIH in Bethesda began to report on the isolation of a retrovirus associated with AIDS. In 1984, many scientists were convinced that the two isolates were the same virus and that the virus was the cause of AIDS (Gallo and Montagnier 1989).

Studies of Behavior Change

Since 1978, investigators from CDC (including later task force members) have been working very closely with investigators in the San Francisco Department of Health on a series of studies of hepatitis B virus infection in 6,700 homosexual and bisexual men (Schreeder et al. 1982). Serum samples drawn from study participants were retrieved from storage and tested for antibody to HIV with the consent of patients after enzyme-linked immunoassays for HIV were developed. Results showed that about 2 percent of study participants were infected in 1978, but we estimate that by now at least 71 percent of these men have been infected with HIV (Byers et al. 1988).

More than 1,300 members of this San Francisco City Clinic Cohort were interviewed at enrollment in 1978, 1979, or 1980 and again in 1984 or later. During this time, the mean number of reported unprotected receptive anal exposures with ejaculation

Figure 6.11. AIDS Information in San Francisco

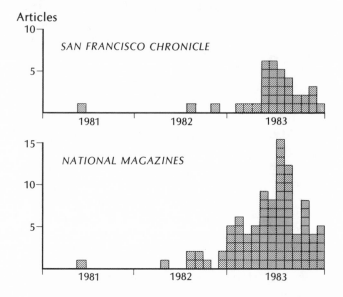

Figure 6.12. Percent of Never-Married Women, 15-19 Years Old, Who Have Had Sexual Intercourse, United States

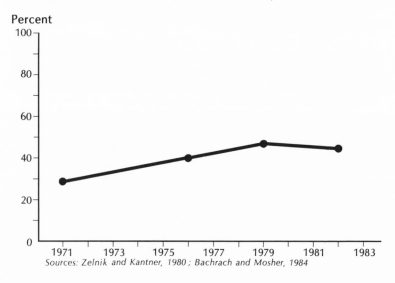

Sources: Zelnik and Kantner, 1980 ; Bachrach and Mosher, 1984

Table 6.1. HIV Prevalence among Female Prostitutes in the U.S.

Study site	IV-drug use number seropositive/ number tested (%)	No IV-drug use number seropositive/ number tested (%)	Total number seropositive/ number tested (%)
Southern Nevada	0/10 (0)	0/27 (0)	0/37 (0)
Atlanta	1/65 (1.5)	0/58 (0)	1/123 (0.8)
Colorado Springs	2/52 (3.8)	0/46 (0)	2/98 (2.0)
Los Angeles	6/163 (3.7)	6/137 (4.4)	12/300 (4.0)
San Francisco	10/101 (9.9)	0/111 (0)	10/212 (4.7)
Miami	46/173 (26.6)	20/267 (7.5)	66/440 (15.0)
Southern New Jersey	6/14 (42.9)	0/14 (0)	6/28 (21.4)
Northern New Jersey	67/115 (58.3)	8/43 (18.6)	75/158 (47.5)
Total	138/693 (19.9)	34/703 (4.8)	172/1,396 (12.3)

Source: Darrow et al. 1990

by nonsteady partners in the four months before interview fell from fifteen in 1978 to less than one in 1986 (Darrow 1988). This is the most convincing evidence that we have for dramatic changes in the sexual practices of homosexual and bisexual men in a major U.S. city.

Changes in sexual practices could have occurred for a number of reasons. Although the media did not immediately respond to reports of cases in 1981, media attention to AIDS began to pick up in 1983, just before we reinterviewed participants in our longitudinal study (figure 6.11).

Data from a series of cross-sectional studies of never-married women 15–19 years old living in households in the United States showed that the proportion engaging in sexual intercourse increased in the 1970s (Zelnik and Kantner 1980), and then leveled off or declined slightly (Bachrach and Mosher 1984) (figure 6.12). No national data are available on the sexual behavior patterns of a representative sample of young women between 1982 and 1988, but data from the 1988 National Survey of Family Growth are now being analyzed at the National Center for Health Statistics and should be available soon. A recently completed study of never-married men 17–19 years old living in metropolitan areas of the United States shows that the proportion engaging in sexual intercourse increased by 15 percent between 1979 and 1988, but condom use at last intercourse increased from 21 percent in 1979 to 58 percent in 1988 (Sonenstein, Pleck, and Ku 1989).

Studies of Heterosexual Transmission

CDC is collaborating with other investigators in a three-phase study of prostitutes and their sexual and needle-sharing partners in an attempt to understand the social dynamics of prostitution and the spread of HIV (Darrow et al. 1989). The objectives of the first phase were to assess the seroprevalence of HIV antibody in prostitute women working in eight different areas of the United States and to identify risks for HIV infection (table 6.1). Overall, 12.3 percent of 1,396 women tested were HIV-antibody positive, but rates ranged from zero among brothel workers in southern Nevada to 47.5 percent among street prostitutes in northern New Jersey (Darrow et al. 1990). Prostitutes with histories of intravenous (IV) drug use were four times more likely to be infected with HIV than those with no evidence of IV-drug use (19.9 percent vs. 4.8 percent). Nevertheless IV-drug use did not appear to be a risk factor for HIV infection in Los Angeles.

Phase II studies are now under way. In Colorado Springs, for example, we are attempting to study the social networks of female prostitutes in an effort to see how women who exchange sexual services for money are linked to other groups by their social, sexual, and drug-using activities (Klovdahl 1985) (figure 6.13). Preliminary findings suggest that over half of the women enrolled in this prospective study have histories of IV-drug use, and the few who are infected with HIV have shared needles or syringes. To date, no HIV infections in female prostitutes or their clients can be directly linked to sexual exposures.

In Phase III, we intend to implement a series of planned interventions to determine if behaviors can be changed to reduce or eliminate risks of HIV transmission to those who might be placing themselves or others at risk of HIV infection. In San

Figure 6.13. Linkage of High-Risk Groups in Colorado Springs, Colorado

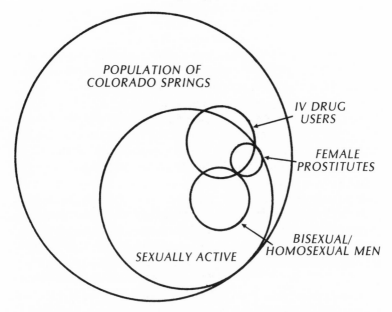

Figure 6.14. AIDS in Areas with <50,000 Residents*

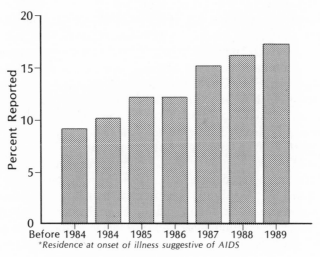

*Residence at onset of illness suggestive of AIDS

Francisco, for example, the California Prostitutes Education Project has produced educational materials and conducted workshops to promote "safer sex" (Alexander 1988). We would like to evaluate the effectiveness of this approach in preventing further spread of HIV and other STDs.

In our research projects, we provide information to and answer the questions of study participants after we gather information from them about their personal experiences. We encourage prostitutes and their sex and needle-sharing partners to be tested for HIV and other STDs and to obtain test results and receive treatment for any abnormalities detected. We also encourage drug users to enroll in drug treatment programs.

Most of the educational and prevention programs now being implemented in the United States are looking at the cognitive, social, and environmental influences on behaviors associated with HIV disease. However, emotional or affective considerations may also be important. Preliminary data suggest that personal experiences with a person with AIDS significantly facilitate behavior change (McKusick et al. 1985).

Recent reports from CDC suggest that HIV is spreading from coastal urban areas to less populated areas of the United States and infecting more racial and ethnic minorities (Centers for Disease Control 1990b). Before 1984, 9 percent of reported AIDS cases were among residents of areas with less than 50,000 population; now 17 percent of reported cases are in such areas (figure 6.14). The ten areas with more than 100 AIDS cases (as of October 1, 1989) and fewer than 50,000 residents were an interesting combination of small towns (table 6.2). At the top of the list was rural Belle Glade in southern Florida, where almost all the people with AIDS were black heterosexual men and women who had worked as migrant farm laborers (Castro et al. 1988). Following Belle Glade were two well-recognized gay enclaves— Key West, Florida, and West Hollywood, California. North Fort Myers, Florida, was next with a significant number of black homosexual men reported with AIDS. The next towns, Decatur, Georgia, and Plainfield, New Jersey, had large numbers of AIDS cases in black heterosexual men and women. Two more gay enclaves, Laguna Beach and exclusive Palm Springs, followed. Sing Sing prison accounted for most of the cases in

**Table 6.2. AIDS in Areas with < 50,000 Population and
>100 Cases, October 1, 1989**

Place	Total number	Black	Hispanic	Heterosexual
			Percentage	
Belle Glade, Fla.	245	98.4	1.2	77.1
Key West, Fla.	214	6.5	1.9	4.2
W. Hollywood, Calif.	176	2.8	9.7	0.6
N. Fort Meyers, Fla.	164	55.5	1.2	49.4
Decatur, Ga.	127	54.3	0.8	17.3
Plainfield, N.J.	116	75.9	7.8	64.7
Laguna Beach, Calif.	115	0.9	6.1	0.9
Palm Springs, Calif.	109	0.9	6.4	1.8
Ossining, N.Y.	107	37.4	39.3	88.8
Hoboken, N.J.	102	7.8	46.1	48.1

the next town, Ossining, New York, but a large proportion of
Hispanic-Americans reported with AIDS were living across the
Hudson River from New York City in Hoboken, New Jersey.

Conclusion

Since the first cases of AIDS were recognized in 1981, social
scientists, epidemiologists, and other researchers have been
working together to formulate and answer questions about the
origin and evolution of the HIV epidemic. In the early years of
the epidemic, 1981 to 1984, scientific attention focused on two
questions: what is the cause of AIDS, and how does it spread
through a population? The answers were that a previously unrecognized retrovirus is the cause and that it is transmitted from
an infected person to a susceptible person during unprotected
sexual exposures, through needle or syringe sharing, or by
direct contact, transfusion, or infusion with contaminated blood
or blood products.

As evidence supporting the hypothesis of a sexually transmitted or blood-borne infectious agent emerged from socioepidemiologic studies, guidelines for the protection of the blood
supply and recommendations for the prevention of sexual transmission of HIV were formulated, debated, and adopted. A sero-

logic test for antibody to HIV was approved in 1985 to screen potential blood donors and to test persons concerned about their health for evidence of HIV infection. The San Francisco City Clinic cohort study of hepatitis B in homosexual and bisexual men also offered the HIV antibody test to participants. Results from the study indicated that HIV had spread extensively among persons who engaged in certain behaviors, such as unprotected receptive anal intercourse with an HIV-antibody-positive partner or with large numbers of partners, some of whom might have been infected with HIV.

Intervention programs were quickly developed to inform persons of the risks of HIV infection associated with specific behaviors and to encourage and reinforce behavior change. Among members of the San Francisco City Clinic cohort interviewed in 1978, 1979, or 1980 and again in 1984 or later, dramatic reductions in self-reported, high-risk sexual activities were observed. These changes apparently resulted from a combination of factors, including information obtained through formal and informal channels, personal experiences with HIV disease or with persons with AIDS, and a recognition that norms governing acceptable sexual contact must change through collective action.

Local, national, and global HIV prevention programs are continually being developed, implemented, and evaluated for persons who remain at risk for acquiring HIV or transmitting it to others. Included among these persons are men who have sex with men but do not identify themselves as being at risk, intravenous drug users who are not enrolled in drug detoxification or treatment programs, the spouses and other sex partners of HIV-infected persons, and sexually active HIV-infected women who are unaware of their serostatus and the risk of transmitting their infection to their infants should they become pregnant. Seroepidemiologic studies, such as the three-phase study of female prostitutes and their sex- and needle-sharing partners described in this chapter, have been designed to determine how some of these persons at risk can be reached, enrolled in research-intervention-evaluation studies, and influenced to modify their behaviors associated with HIV infection and transmission.

Many questions remain about the future course of the HIV epidemic and how the risks for further transmission can be minimized or eliminated. Intervention activities—such as targeted risk-reduction messages delivered by peers through community-based and national minority organizations, personal counseling and voluntary HIV-antibody testing to initiate behavior change, and partner notification and referral—are being carefully examined and reexamined to assure that the most culturally sensitive, cost-effective, and beneficial mix of services is provided to each target group. Lessons learned from the continuing serosurveillance of the HIV epidemic, surveys of behavior change in populations at risk, and evaluations of the impact and outcome of intervention activities should serve to guide policy in the 1990s.

Scientific research can only be conducted in a social system that is willing to take a critical look at itself. AIDS has forced us to examine certain previously ignored aspects of social life. In the 1990s, social as well as other scientists will be given opportunities to contribute to the development and evaluation of more effective methods for preventing the transmission of HIV in the United States and elsewhere.

7

An Anthropological Research Agenda for an AIDS Epicenter within the United States

RONALD STALL

The purpose of this chapter is to outline potential anthropological contributions to a research agenda used by the Behavioral Medicine Component of the Center for AIDS Prevention Studies (CAPS) at the University of California, San Francisco to organize the development of new research projects (Coates, Temoshok, and Mandel 1984; Coates et al. 1986). The chapter will begin by describing the research agenda and the Behavioral Medicine component at CAPS. Second, an example of the applications of the research agenda within the city of San Francisco will be given. The balance of the chapter will outline how medical anthropology can be used to extend this research agenda.

A Psychosocial Research Agenda for the Study of AIDS

Since the earliest days of the American experience with AIDS, health researchers and the lay public have shown strong interest in the psychosocial aspects of HIV infection. This interest has been focused primarily on the responses of the disparate social groups in which the AIDS epidemic initially concentrated and on the effects of psychosocial factors on the onset of AIDS within infected persons. Early in the epidemic, Coates, Temoshok, and Mandel (1984) present a psychosocial research agenda for AIDS that included four major components:

(1) *Primary Prevention.* The first of the four components

concerns understanding how to motivate individuals to lower risk for the transmission of HIV. This includes measuring the prevalence of specific high-risk behaviors as well as determining the correlates of risk-taking behavior for HIV infection. Of particular interest within this agenda is the identification of circumstances under which individuals are more likely to engage in high-risk behaviors for the transmission of HIV. The study of subpopulations at especially high risk for HIV transmission—minorities, adolescents and young adults, substance abusers, people who relapse from safe sex—falls under this component of the research agenda.

(2) *Secondary Prevention.* The second of the components involves understanding the impact of psychosocial variables on disease incidence and progression. This research focus is designed to determine whether psychosocial variables are implicated in the progression of HIV disease. If relationships between psychosocial variables and disease progression are found, interventions can be designed that may delay clinical manifestations of HIV disease. Understanding the distinctions between those HIV-infected persons who "comply" with prescribed AIDS drug prophylactics or who undertake "early intervention" and those HIV-infected persons who do not is also relevant to this body of research. Such interventions constitute secondary prevention, the prevention of onset of frank illness among those already infected with HIV.

(3) *Understanding How to Provide Care.* The third of the research components concerns understanding the psychosocial impact of the HIV disease process itself. Selected topics of interest under this component include the psychosocial consequences of HIV disease diagnosis on the individual, understanding the condition under which individuals are able to elicit care for HIV disease, the impact of the epidemic within specific communities, and the effects of the epidemic on caregivers.

(4) *Evaluation.* The final component of the agenda concerns evaluating the efficacy of various AIDS prevention strategies. Based on understandings concerning the conditions under which high risk behavior occurs, interventions can be designed to lower rates of behaviors that can transmit HIV. As already mentioned, the prevalence studies can also be used to identify

subpopulations at especially high risk so that specialized interventions can be designed for these populations.

Two years after the original Coates, Temeoshok, and Mandel review, Coates et al. (1986) reviewed the existing literature to determine whether this research agenda had been supported by empirical evidence. They found, even after that short two-year period, that considerable empirical evidence had accumulated from across the United States and Europe to demonstrate the effects of psychosocial factors on shaping the AIDS epidemic.

The conclusions of the Coates et al. (1986) review regarding the state of the psychosocial AIDS literature still stand: there is considerable evidence to support the contention that an understanding of psychosocial factors is central to the prevention of risky behaviors for the transmission of HIV. A much smaller literature has measured the effects of behavioral, psychological, or social variables on the progression of HIV disease. A growing literature has emerged that describes psychosocial sequelae among distinct groups of persons diagnosed at different stages of HIV disease, as well as the effects of the epidemic on specific communities and caregivers. Finally, a nascent literature has appeared to describe the effects of different interventions that attempt to prevent risky behavior for HIV transmission or modify the natural history of HIV disease.

The Behavioral Medicine Component at the Center for AIDS Prevention Studies is composed of a group of several social psychologists and social/behavioral scientists. The origins of the group can be traced to the initiation of the AIDS Behavioral Research Project, a long-term, ongoing cohort study of risk-taking and care-seeking behaviors of gay-identified men in San Francisco, although most of the members of the component had previously conducted research on risk-taking behaviors for other diseases or chronic conditions. Research efforts within the component are highly collegial—a strong emphasis is placed on collaboration and cross-fertilization of ideas. Little emphasis is placed on disciplinary affiliations, and no positions are allocated to members of particular disciplines. Investigators are free to pursue their own interests and now have available to them several large AIDS data sets for analysis.

The Epidemiological Context of the Research Agenda

AIDS RISK REDUCTIONS AMONG SELF-IDENTIFIED GAY MEN. Changes in sexual risk for HIV infection made by self-identified gay men in San Francisco from 1984 to 1987 have been observed in two independent prospective cohorts over that time period—the AIDS Behavioral Research Project (ABRP) and the Communication Technologies (CT) Surveys. Study of the behavioral responses made by gay men to the AIDS epidemic has generally been complicated by sampling problems. These sampling limitations derive from the fact that it is probably impossible in practice to enumerate the total population of men who have sex with other men residing within a given political boundary. These two studies undertook to sample self-identified gay men in San Francisco over the same period of time. Comparison of the behavioral changes manifested within both of these cohorts provides a test of the validity of the observed changes within both cohorts. Although there have been several published studies describing changes in high-risk sexual behavior among gay men in San Francisco, this is the first report to compare long-term trends across two different samples of gay men, to summarize these trends for a four-year period, and to extend the description of trends in risk reduction into the recent past.

Both the ABRP and CT surveys sampled the gay male community of San Francisco in different ways, thereby providing independent perspectives on the behavioral adaptations of gay men to the AIDS epidemic. Given this sampling variation, considerable confidence can be placed in observed trends replicated across the two studies. Both samples have also used the same time period (one month) for the measurement of sexual risk. Although use of this one-month window of measurement has been consistent across the two studies, the question arises as to whether a one-month measurement period is a representative measure of sexual risk taken across the previous year. Use of longer time periods of measurement for sexual risk, on the other hand, may also introduce bias because of respondent recall error. The principal investigators of both studies independently concluded that a one-month measurement period was likely to maximize reliability, while recognizing that there might be some loss in the representativeness of respondents' sexual patterns over time.

The ABRP was originally designed to determine how the AIDS epidemic was influencing gay men's psychological adjustment and sexual risk behavior. As one of the first behavioral surveys of gay male risk behavior in the nation, it has provided the empirical basis for a number of papers describing the prevalence and predictors of risk within this population (Stall et al. 1986; Coates, et al. 1986). A survey questionnaire has been administered to the cohort semiannually from November 1983 until November 1986 and annually thereafter. The convenience sample was initially obtained by soliciting bathhouse and bar patrons, men who found their sexual partners through neither baths nor bars, and male couples, for an overall response rate of 51 percent. Taking convenience samples from relatively distinct subgroups of gay men was undertaken to maximize the potential for constructing a balanced picture of the types of changes in sexual behavior that gay men in general have made in response to the AIDS epidemic. This method of recruitment resulted in an initial group of participants with higher overall numbers of sexual partners than were found in two separate samples of gay men in San Francisco, particularly for men not involved in relationships.

As of the November 1987 wave of data collection, 76 percent of the original cohort either continued to respond to the survey (70 percent) or were known to have died (6 percent). Although there has been some variation in questionnaire construction from one wave to another, the primary emphasis of the instrument has been to describe the prevalence of risk for HIV infection within the sample and to identify the correlates of this risk. Core items thus include a detailed measure of sexual risk, level of health education and beliefs, recent history of sexually transmitted diseases, a psychological inventory, attitudes about AIDS, adaptations made to the AIDS epidemic and personal experience of the effects of the epidemic, and a series of drug and alcohol items (concerning the combination of drugs/alcohol and sex). There was no statistically significant difference between the original 1984 cohort who were surveyed in 1987 and those who were lost to follow-up in 1987 for time 1 age, relationship status, mutual monogamy, level of sexual risk, and frequency of using condoms during sex.

The San Francisco AIDS Foundation commissioned the first CT Survey in the summer of 1984 to determine how San Francisco's gay and bisexual male population was responding to the AIDS epidemic. The initial survey was designed not only to determine the level of sexual risk within the gay and bisexual male population but also to identify the correlates of high risk sex, to determine the baseline extent of health education knowledge, and to explore which kinds of messages were most likely to induce men to change risky behaviors. Subsequent surveys were commissioned by the San Francisco AIDS Foundation in 1985, 1986, and 1987 to follow trends in risk and correlates of risk over time. Respondents were sampled from a Metromail Corporation list of San Francisco households with listed telephone numbers. The Metromail Corporation constructs a list of households with telephones initially by data drawn from telephone companies; this list is further augmented with data from secondary sources. The secondary sources include voter registration lists, post office change of address forms, insurance lists, and driver's license and vehicle registration data. Augmentation of the list of households with telephones occurs every weekend. Estimates by the Metromail Corporation indicate that their procedures are likely to undersample households that are very wealthy, very poor, or in transition.

Only households listed by initials or by male names were selected for the CT sampling frame, a total of some 9,735 households. Each census tract in the city was assigned a weight representing the proportion of unmarried males residing in that tract. The sample was then drawn according to these weighted proportions. Some 4,772 households were successfully contacted. Of these, 1,444 were composed of women only at the time of the telephone contact, 1,961 had a resident male but not a resident male that self-identified as gay after screening, 529 had a resident gay male, and 838 of the successful contacts refused to undergo either the screening or the interview. It should be noted that of the 838 respondents who refused to undergo interviewing or screening, interviewers coded 696 as "probably not gay men" and 142 as "probably gay men." Of the

529 sample households both containing self-identifying gay or bisexual males and at home when called, 500 respondents (the sample size required by the San Francisco AIDS Foundation) were interviewed. Of the households with resident males, 2,490 agreed to be interviewed, for a response rate of approximately 75 percent. Among the men who either self-identified as gay men or who were coded by the interviewers as "probably gay," 500 were interviewed, again for a response rate of 75 percent. All respondents were at least eighteen years of age and reported having sex with other men at least occasionally or identified themselves as gay or bisexual.

The second wave of data collection (conducted during the spring of 1985) consisted of 300 reinterviews from the first sample wave and 200 additional interviews (drawn from a separate probability sample using the same techniques as for the first wave). The strategy of taking 300 longitudinal interviews with 200 additional interviews was adopted to test for combined sensitization effects of the interview instrument and loss to follow-up bias. This same strategy was adopted for the third and fourth waves of data collection. The third wave (during the spring of 1986) consisted of 236 longitudinal reinterviews with an additional cross-sectional sample (n = 201); the fourth wave consisted of 189 longitudinal interviews with an additional cross-sectional sample of 201. Sampling methods and administration of interviews were consistent across all waves of data collection.

The core set of items consistently asked during the CT Surveys include detailed measures of sexual risk, proximity/ threat of the AIDS epidemic to the respondent, enjoyment of specific sexual practices, beliefs about the comparative pleasures of safe and risky sex, contact with education campaigns, HIV antibody status and beliefs about testing, the combination of drugs and alcohol with sex, and demographics. There were no significant differences between the 1984 CT sample that formed the longitudinal cohort and those men who were not successfully followed in age, ethnicity, income, education, or level of risk for HIV infection. The same comparisons were made between the longitudinal cohort and the new cross-sectional ple drawn in 1987. Of the comparisons listed previously, only age was significantly different in 1987. This difference is to be expected since the longitudinal cohort has aged since originally being drawn, while the new cross-sectional samples can now sample men that were too young to be interviewed in 1984. This explanation for the differences between the longitudinal cohort and the new cross-sectional sample is supported by the fact that the primary differences between the two samples are found in the proportion of men less than thirty years old.

MEASURES OF SEXUAL RISK. Sexual risk for HIV infection was measured during the period of the previous thirty days for both of these research projects. From these ongoing measures, we have replicated, with some modifications, a scale developed by the Chicago Multi-center AIDS Cohort Study (MACS) group that predicts HIV seroconversion over time among gay/bisexual men (Joseph et al. 1987). This scale has four categories. Those at "no risk" are celibate. Those at "low risk" only had anal sex with a condom within the bounds of a monogamous relationship or, if not monogamous, no anal sex at all. Men who fall in the "modified high risk" category only have anal sex without a condom within the bounds of a monogamous relationship or, of not monogamous, only have anal sex while using condoms. Those at "high risk" have anal sex without condoms outside of monogamous relationships. This scale has been modified so that any form of anal sex without a condom is used to define risk group membership, rather than only receptive anal sex without a condom. This modification was made because of the possibility that insertive anal sex is a risk behavior for HIV seroconversion and because from a prevention point of view any form of unprotected anal sex is undesirable.

The scale developed by the Chicago MACS groups is essentially qualitative: it does not quantitatively measure participation in high-risk, sexual activities with nonmonogamous partners. Thus, persons who had only one high-risk sexual encounter are placed in the same category as those who might have such encounters daily. To summarize quantitative risk, I have used a simple summary measure of the number of times each respondent had unprotected anal intercourse with a non-monogamous partner.

FINDINGS.   Table 7.1 demonstrates the prevalence of various levels of sexual risk for HIV infection as measured by the CT Surveys since 1984. As is evident from this table, profound risk reductions have occurred since the first wave of measurement. The prevalence of high-risk sexual behavior dropped from 31 percent on intake to 7 percent by 1987, a 77 percent decline in the prevalence of risk from 1984 to 1987. The modal risk category within this sample was high-risk in 1984, but changed to low-risk by the following year and has remained at that level since that time.

Table 7.2 summarizes the changes that gay men in the AIDS Behavioral Research Project (ABRP) have made since 1984. Although there appear to be differences in the prevalence of certain levels of risk, the overall trends of change observed in this study replicate those found in the CT data. The men in the ABRP evidenced a dramatic decline of 59 percent in participation in high-risk sexual behavior from 1984 to 1987. Further, as had been the case with the CT Surveys, the modal risk level in 1984 for this sample was at high risk but changed to low risk by 1985 and has stayed at that level since that time.

Regarding differences between the two samples, it is clear that the ABRP sample initially sampled more men at high risk and that the high-risk segment of the ABRP has been consistently larger than that found in the CT cohort. It is not surprising that the ABRP has consistently contained a larger subset of gay men who practice high-risk sexual behavior since the ABRP was comprised of a series of opportunistic samples drawn to no small degree from the patrons of bars and bathhouses. In this sense, then, both samples give a complementary perspective on changes in sexual behavior among gay men in San Francisco. The CT Surveys provide a view of trends that are occurring in a household-based sample, while the ABRP contains an oversampling of men who were initially at high risk of HIV transmission.

However, trend analyses are not appropriate to the study of occasional relapse from safe sex techniques. Cross-sectional trend rates for participation in high-risk sex do not measure

**Table 7.1. Change in the Prevalence of Levels of Sexual Risk
for HIV Infection During the Previous 30 Days, 1984-1987,
for Gay and Bisexual Men in San Francisco:
Communication Technology Surveys,
Longitudinal Cohort, Valid Percentages
(N = 189)**

Modified MACS risk scale	Year of measurement			
	1984	1985	1986	1987
No risk	21.9	28.0	28.9	30.3
Low risk	29.9	35.4	36.7	40.4
Modified high risk	17.6	21.7	24.1	22.3
High risk	30.5	13.2	10.2	6.9

**Table 7.2. Change in the Prevalence of Levels of Sexual Risk
for HIV Infection During the Previous 30 Days, 1984-1987,
for Gay and Bisexual Men in San Francisco:
The AIDS Behavioral Research Project,
Longitudinal Cohort, Valid Percentages
(N = 473)**

Modified MACS risk scale	Year of measurement			
	1984	1985	1986	1987
No risk	12.6	16.2	13.8	22.5
Low risk	30.8	39.4	41.7	37.1
Modified high risk	17.9	23.4	25.3	25.0
High risk	38.7	21.1	19.1	15.5

**Table 7.3. Individual Patterns of Change in Participation in
High-Risk Sex for HIV Transmission During the Previous
30 Days, 1984-1987, for Gay and Bisexual Men in San
Francisco: The AIDS Behaviorial Research Project,
Longitudinal Cohort, Valid Percentages
(N = 461; missing data = 12)**

	Percent	n
Stable lower risk	50.3	(232)
Changed to lower risk	29.7	(137)
Relapse	15.9	(75)
Stable high risk	3.6	(17)

individual change over time. Rather, these figures measure levels of risk for HIV transmission for the entire sample at four different points in time. Individual paths of change in risk for HIV transmission from 1984 to 1987 can also be summarized. This analysis will yield estimates of the proportion of men who were a consistent low risk in comparison to the men who had occasionally relapsed from behavioral risk reductions.

These rates were calculated by determining whether an individual respondent for the ABRP was at high risk (as defined earlier) at any one measurement point. This approach results in sixteen different possible individual patterns of change over the four measurement points, all of which were represented in the sample. These sixteen different paths of change were collapsed into four different summary patterns: stable low risk (not at high risk at all four waves), changed to low risk (changed from high risk to low risk without returning to high risk), relapse (changed for at least one wave to high risk from low risk), and stable high risk (at high risk for all four waves). These rates are based on behaviors engaged in during the previous thirty days, and as such they may underestimate or overestimate patterns of sexual risk-taking for an entire year. Summary rates of sexual risk-taking are given in table 7.3.

From table 7.3 it can be seen that 50.3 percent (232 men) fell into the "stable low risk" category, 29.7 percent fell into the "changed to low risk" category, 15.9 percent fell into the "relapse" category, and 3.6 percent fell into the "stable high risk" category. Thus, the pattern of relapse is four times more common over time than that of consistent high-risk sex. Given the very high background rates of HIV infection within this community during this time period, it is clear that relapses from safe sex, however occasional, constitute a threat to the health of gay men in San Francisco.

These findings replicate and expand over time the data from other reports (Winkelstein et al. 1987) that have periodically described changes in sexual risk for HIV infection made by gay and bisexual men in San Francisco in response to the AIDS epidemic. The descriptions given here support the widespread impression that profound behavioral risk reductions have occurred within this community since the early 1980s.

Notably, data from both the AIDS Behavioral Research Project (ABRP) and the Communication Technologies (CT) studies indicate that the trends in reduced sexual risk for HIV infection, already documented by the mid-1980s, are continuing. It appears that the possibility of new HIV infection among gay men in San Francisco continues to decline over time. Thus, the behavior changes described here are among the most profound noted in the public health literature and do not appear to be subject on a widespread basis to relapse. These findings stand in considerable contrast to the literatures regarding other life-threatening health-related behaviors, such as drug or alcohol abuse, anorexia nervosa, tobacco smoking, or dietary intake of cholesterol, in which initial behavioral risk reduction has not been as widespread and yet relapse from the behavioral changes that do occur appears to be much more common. Nonetheless, relapse from safe sex appears to be considerably more common than consistent high-risk sex, implying that prevention campaigns will now have to take this form of sexual risk-taking into account.

HEALTH CARE IMPLICATIONS OF AIDS IN SAN FRANCISCO. San Francisco has already suffered staggering losses as a result of the AIDS epidemic. As Mayor Art Agnos pointed out in testimony to the Presidential Commission on AIDS (1988), San Francisco has already lost twice as many men to the AIDS epidemic as were lost from that city during World War I, World War II, the Korean War, and the Vietnam War combined (Agnos, 1988). The numbers of men likely to be diagnosed with AIDS in the near future are widely expected to burden the local health care system until it approaches the breaking point. Finding the means to provide care to those likely to be diagnosed with AIDS over the next five years has become an issue of genuine concern (Baker and Moulton 1988), particularly as the time of survival after diagnosis with AIDS lengthens. It should also be mentioned that the prevalence of HIV infection in San Francisco— about 5 percent of the total adult population— approaches that of many African urban centers. Describing how this epidemic is likely to affect a wealthy city of the industrialized West gives a chilling forecast of the effects to be felt in parts of the Third World.

Baker and Moulton (1988) have attempted to estimate the effects of the epidemic within the gay community and the wider city through 1993. As widely observed, the epidemic in San Francisco has centered among gay and bisexual men. By 1993, it is estimated that about 92 percent of resident San Franciscans with AIDS will be drawn from within the male gay/bisexual community. And even as late as 1993, about 86 percent of those infected with HIV will be gay men. It is currently estimated, from one long-term natural history study of HIV infection, that approximately 50 percent of the gay male population in San Francisco is currently infected with HIV (Winkelstein et al. 1987). Cumulative prevalence of HIV infection in a subset of another cohort (defined for a Hepatitis B vaccine trial) rose from 1 percent in 1978 to 46.3 percent by mid-1987 (Hessol et al. 1988). From this same cohort we know that the majority of the seroconversions occurred during the years 1980 through 1982, with 15 percent seroconverting during the peak year of 1982. The seroconversion rate then fell dramatically to 5 percent in 1983 and subsequently declined to less than 1 percent in 1986 and has stayed at that level since that time (see also Winkelstein et al. 1987). In short, the majority of the infections among gay and bisexual men happened well before the first clinical manifestations of AIDS appeared among gay men and long before the isolation of HIV as the cause of AIDS.

By combining the historical cumulative rise of prevalence of HIV infection among gay men in San Francisco with observed rates of progression to full-blown AIDS over time, estimates can be made of the rates of future diagnoses and deaths through the early 1990s. For example, Lemp et al. (1988) have estimated that the number of San Franciscans diagnosed with AIDS will fall between 12,349 and 17,022 by mid-1993. As it is expected that 92 percent of these cases will be drawn from among gay or bisexual men, the toll within that community can also be estimated. Taking the mid-point of these estimates (14,686) and applying the expected proportion of diagnoses drawn from among gay or bisexual men (92 percent) yields a figure of some 13,511 cases. The San Francisco Department of Public Health estimates that some 55,816 resident San Franciscans are gay men, suggesting that approximately one out of every four men currently resident in San Francisco will either be diagnosed with or dead from AIDS by mid-1993.

Given a socio-medical catastrophe of such dimensions, the primary AIDS research priority must concern prevention: nearly half of San Francisco's gay men remain uninfected with HIV, although continued HIV seroconversion still exists (Lifson, Stall, and Winkelstein 1989). Further prevention of new infections among needle users and their heterosexual contacts is an urgent priority. Prevention, in the case of AIDS, means the modification of behaviors strongly shaped by cultural factors and which occur well beyond the reach of governmental regulatory agencies. Secondary prevention (the prevention of the onset of clinical symptoms of AIDS) may turn out to be a central prevention effort if it is shown that behavioral variables are implicated as co-factors for AIDS disease progression or, perhaps more likely, if it is shown that psychosocial variables impact on the decision to pursue early clinical interventions for HIV infection.

Another important research agenda within San Francisco concerns the clinical care of those infected with HIV. San Francisco has developed a much-copied model of AIDS care that is fueled to no small degree by volunteer care labor provided from within the community and provided outside of hospital walls. The willingness of San Franciscans to continue to provide many thousands of hours of volunteer care has contributed in important ways to lowering the costs of caring for persons with AIDS (Arno 1987). However, the question of whether a city's population can continue to volunteer low-technology medical care if one-fourth of a large community within that city is sick or dead has not yet been answered. Effective models of care delivery for persons with AIDS that do not depend on expensive hospital-based labor must be found. Understanding the psychosocial consequences of HIV infection and/or an AIDS diagnosis is necessary to providing humane and cost-effective care to persons with HIV infection. Identifying the conditions under which persons can continue to provide care in the face of a horrifying epidemic will prove essential to maintaining adequate levels of professional and lay caregivers. Finally, evaluation of methods to meet all of these goals will prove to be an essential tool.

Thus far, I have primarily discussed psychosocial research in terms of the needs of gay men, the group in San Francisco with the highest prevalence rates of HIV infection and the group that has suffered the highest cumulative incidence of AIDS. However, it is also important to point out that goals of this research agenda also address the needs of separate populations at risk: needle users, ethnic minorities, adolescents, and others. Thus, the goals of this research agenda are directly relevant to the needs imposed by the AIDS epidemic in San Francisco and in other North American epicenters across disparate populations at high risk of HIV transmission.

The Uses of Anthropology in an American AIDS Epicenter

Anthropological research techniques are especially well-suited to broadening understandings of the AIDS epidemic for several reasons. First, one of the distinctive aspects of the AIDS epidemic has been its manifestation within remarkably different subpopulations, each of which is characterized by distinct combinations of behaviors implicated in the spread of HIV infection. For this reason, the AIDS epidemic can be thought of as a series of subepidemics, each with its own set of challenges for prevention and management. Thus, the circumstances under which urban gay men take risks for HIV infection are not the same as those of ethnic minority needle users, nor are the reasons for risk-taking in these two groups the same as among African women in Rwanda. It also goes without saying that the challenges faced by these three groups and others in obtaining effective health care once symptoms of HIV infection emerge are going to be distinct. Since the epidemic has manifested itself in such diverse cultural groups, an understanding of how culture shapes risk-taking and care-seeking behaviors will be necessary in the worldwide fight against AIDS.

Although it has been known for some time that AIDS has a worldwide distribution, prevention theorists are just beginning to face up to the reality that the epidemic will have to be fought across cultures. Primary prevention, in the case of HIV transmission, involves modifying intimate and commonplace behaviors that are governed by different constraints across

cultures. Prevention workers must have a good working knowledge of cultures at risk of widespread HIV transmission if their
efforts are to be effective. Although it will hardly be news to an
anthropologist that risk reduction interventions that work
among urban gay men cannot be assumed to meet with success
in Uganda, the first instinct of many AIDS prevention workers
will be to try and modify the successful AIDS prevention efforts
found to be effective in the West for use in Africa or (more
commonly) to attempt to modify prevention strategies that have
worked for middle-class whites to ethnic minorities or drug
addicts. Anthropology is the primary behavioral science that
can provide the descriptive information concerning the cultural
factors that define risky needle use or sexual practices so that
prevention efforts can be intelligently designed across cultures
or distinct populations.

Second, the concentration of AIDS among a set of stigmatized or minority populations in the West has meant that
sampling of those at greatest risk of HIV infection is difficult.
These well-recognized sampling difficulties mean that the standard ethnographic methods used to reach respondents are no
more likely to result in sampling bias than are the opportunistic
sampling methods employed by most AIDS survey researchers.
Third, measurement of risk for HIV infection has almost entirely depended on respondent recall for periods of as long as a
year. Given the enormous potential for bias because of respondent recall problems, the observation of respondents in their
natural settings becomes a compelling selling point for ethnographic research proposals. It should also be pointed out that
findings from survey data are often difficult to interpret, particularly if researchers do not have a good working understanding of the population under study or are not themselves
members of that community. It is useless, for example, to attempt to interpret the finding that "nonwhite ethnicity" is
associated with greater risk for HIV transmission without a
good ethnographic understanding of the particular groups
being described. Finally, current theory that describes "noncompliance" has been almost entirely developed through the
study of white middle-class populations. There has been relatively little research on the special considerations of ethnic

minorities or intravenous drug users concerning "noncompliance" with health education messages in general or, more specifically, the factors surrounding behavior risk-taking for HIV transmission. Each of these characteristics of the AIDS epidemic and the psychosocial literature support the use of anthropological methods in studying risk-taking behaviors for HIV transmission.

PRIMARY PREVENTION OF HIV INFECTION. At present, the prevention literature is dominated by a body of research based on survey research methods. Survey methods have documented profound behavioral changes among gay men and have been used to identify a set of variables associated with continued risk-taking behaviors (see Becker and Joseph 1988; Joseph et al. 1987; Stall, Coates, and Hoff 1988; Stall and Paul 1989). Variables found to be correlated with sexual risk-taking include the belief that social norms have changed so that unsafe sex is now deviant (O'Reilly et al. 1989), the use of alcohol or drugs during sexual activity (Stall et al. 1986; Stall and Ostrow 1989), personal efficacy (Charles 1985), HIV antibody testing (Coates et al. 1988), and a set of demographic variables. More recently, an attempt has been made to organize both existent health behavior change theory and empirical AIDS data into a unified theory of AIDS risk-taking behavior (Catania, Kegeles, and Coates, in press).

Despite the existence of this developing quantitative literature, there is a pressing need for inductive theory building, based on empirical ethnographic observation/interviews, to explain AIDS risk-taking for groups at high risk of HIV infection. Quantitative analyses must proceed on the basis of variables defined at the onset of a research project and cannot be changed to reflect hypotheses developed after a questionnaire is finalized. Many of the variables initially hypothesized to correlate with AIDS behavioral risk have been derived from existent theory (notably the health belief model). The sole reliance on deductive research designs precludes discovery of variables that respondents may consider crucial in explaining behavior but that may not be suggested by existent behavior change theory or previous research. Closing the exploration of new variables important to risk-taking is premature without an inductive study of the reasons that respondents themselves give for taking risks for HIV transmission. The potential contributions of inductive theory building within a developing field of scientific inquiry cannot be underestimated.

Thus, what is needed at this point in the development of our understanding of risk-taking behaviors for HIV infection is a set of studies that inductively identify, based on qualitative interview data, the factors that promote or inhibit the consistent adherence to AIDS risk reduction messages. Such research should be defined not only to help interpret survey data but also to elicit new reasons for engaging in or not engaging in those behaviors known to facilitate HIV infection. The use of a methodologically-independent approach to understanding risk for HIV transmission should work to expand, replicate, and provide an interpretative context for findings drawn from survey research. This dualist approach should be used across groups at risk—needle users, ethnic minorities, adolescents—to better understand the reasons for taking risks for HIV transmission across disparate populations. At present, few studies have attempted to use qualitative techniques to study risk-taking behavior.

CO-FACTORS FOR HIV DISEASE PROGRESSION. One of the many interesting questions regarding the AIDS epidemic is whether psychosocial or behavioral factors influence the onset of full-blown AIDS symptoms or length of survival after diagnosis. The efficacy of psychosocial or behavioral factors in facilitating disease progression is taken as a matter of faith by many HIV advocacy groups, although few empirical studies have directly tested co-factor hypotheses (see Kaslow et al. 1989). Resolving this question will prove to be a formidable epidemiological task, requiring cooperative analyses of natural history data by psychologists, immunologists, neurologists, epidemiologists, and biostatisticians. The analysis of these data sets does not require uniquely anthropological approaches, with the possible exception of the study of genetic factors on HIV disease progression.

UNDERSTANDING HOW TO CARE FOR PEOPLE WITH AIDS OR HIV INFECTION. Diagnosis with AIDS or of HIV infection sets off a series of important psychosocial consequences. The most immediate of these is the interpretation that the individual places on what is generally regarded as a terrifying medical diagnosis. Interpretations of the news that one is seropositive or has been given an AIDS diagnosis can range from acceptance of the biomedical model to the political (as exemplified by ACT UP organizations) to quasireligious (as exemplified by New Age treatment approaches to HIV infection) or varying mixtures of interpretations.

Decisions must also be made on how to handle, within one's intimate social networks, news that can permanently change important relationships. This is particularly the case when the previous presentation of self did not include a frank admission that the individual engaged in behaviors that can transmit HIV infection. Differing interpretations of the meaning of HIV seropositivity or of news that one is manifesting advanced symptoms of infection can have important implications for the types of care that patients seek. How the diagnosed individual resolves presentation of self issues and/or interprets being infected with HIV may influence in important ways the types of care that the patient seeks (Moulton et al. 1987) or, indeed, the decision to seek health care at all. These decisions can be expected to have very important consequences in terms of lengthening survival after infection if the antiviral drugs and medications to prevent onset of opportunistic infections continue to become more efficacious.

As previously mentioned, in large American epicenters, the number of persons likely to be diagnosed with AIDS over the next decade shows every sign of becoming an intractable sociomedical problem. At present, models of care for persons with AIDS rely on a mix of volunteer and professional care. By relying on low-technology volunteer care, AIDS patients minimize the use of expensive hospital-based care. However, when a health care system must rely on volunteer labor, the possibility exists that different kinds of patients may not be equally, or effectively, served. In order to provide humane and cost-effective care, the needs of persons with AIDS, the demands that they place on the health care system, and the support that they receive outside of the formal care network must be understood.

In order to describe the processes by which different kinds of persons with AIDS access medical care, Stall, Heurtin-Roberts,

Moulton, and Paul are undertaking to describe the differential patterns of seeking and obtaining health care among gay men, intravenous drug users, and their respective cancer controls. This research design is outlined below:

"Designing a Model of Care for
Intravenous Drug Users with AIDS"

AIDS Cases	*Cancer Controls*
Gay men	Men with cancer
Male IVDUs	Men with cancer

This project was designed to describe how intravenous drug users (IVDUs) with AIDS search for and obtain care. By identifying and understanding the behavioral patterns characteristic of IVDUs with AIDS, a cost-effective and human model of health care delivery can be developed to meet the needs of this specialized but large population of patients. In particular it is important to understand how the needs and demands that these patients place on the health care system are different from those of other kinds of AIDS patients, as well as the cancer controls. Thus, this research project is designed to determine what is different about having AIDS from having another life-threatening illness, as well as the differences between gay men with AIDS and intravenous drug users with AIDS.

The research adopted a case-control design, a standard approach to epidemiological research. To identify patterns that are unique to male IVDUs with AIDS, comparison will be made with gay male AIDS patients. Together, these groups of AIDS patients will be compared to cancer patients, a group diagnosed with a disease that could result in a terminal outcome, matched on the basis of age and ethnicity. Excess difference among the three groups of AIDS patients beyond the variables controlled for by the matching strategy can be attributed to the effects of the AIDS diagnosis within that particular risk group. This design has been adopted so that the independent effects of an AIDS diagnosis not attributable to confounding socioeconomic variables are identified.

A primary objective in the construction of the research design has been to construct a set of interview protocols that combines the standardization of quantitative interviews yet also yields a rich body of detail typical of ethnographic interviews. For this research, the interview instrument combined a mix of closed and open-ended items. The quantitative data will be analyzed through the use of deductive statistical methods; the qualitative date will be subjected to an inductive analysis so that discovery of adaptive behaviors made by IVDUs will be maximized. In this manner the two primary objectives of the research project will be met: to show what is different about these groups of patients all diagnosed with a life-threatening illness and to determine respondent-identified reasons for any differences in behaviors and attitudes that may exist. These findings will be related to health policy and treatment issues relevant to the needs of IVDUs with AIDS. This design can be used in the comparison of many different populations in search of care for HIV-related complaints. Further, there is no reason why this design could not be applied to the study of the care needs and social adaptations of persons with subclinical manifestations of HIV infection.

In addition to understanding the needs of persons with AIDS, it is also important to understand how individuals are able to care for persons with HIV infection. What are the conditions under which individuals are able to extend care to others battling a painful and stigmatizing illness? What kinds of support are needed for those who provide care to persons with AIDS? Are burnout rates higher among those who provide care to AIDS patients, and if so, why? How does caring for a person with AIDS affect the caregiver? What are the differences between those who are able to extend care "successfully" and those who find extending such care to be a terrible burden? What is it like to care for a person with AIDS when the caregiver is himself infected with HIV? How do individuals cope who have provided care serially to several individuals with AIDS?

The AIDS epidemic has manifested itself among many disparate populations, resulting in many different kinds of demands upon the health care system in coping with this epidemic. Further, the political economics of health care delivery in the United States has dictated that in the large epicenters, relying on a mix of volunteer and professional care has become necessary. In order to provide cost-effective and humane care, the needs of those battling HIV infection must be understood. Further, understanding the conditions under which individuals can volunteer care (or continue to provide paid professional care) in the face of a horrifying epidemic has also become necessary.

The sole reliance upon quantitative, deductive research methods in meeting these goals would almost certainly be counterproductive. The use of deductive methods requires that questionnaires be constructed on the basis of existing theory. The case can be made that the AIDS epidemic is qualitatively different from the other epidemics historically experienced by Americans, making the sole use of existent theory suspect. The use of qualitative, inductive theory construction is required if we are to understand the conditions under which cost-effective and humane care can be given to those who suffer from HIV infection. For this reason, anthropology can make important contributions to formulating an effective public health response to the AIDS epidemic.

EVALUATION. Evaluation research can be used to determine the effectiveness of both primary and secondary AIDS intervention efforts, as well as to determine the consequences of adopting different kinds of care strategies. Thus, the first task of evaluation is to determine if specific prevention or care strategies have a differential effect in lowering risk, preventing onset of frank illness, saving money, raising satisfaction with care, or requiring less paid labor. Each of these questions can be adequately answered through the use of standard evaluation designs and quantitative data analysis and do not require specialized anthropological contributions.

The second task of evaluation research, however, is to determine why specific interventions have the outcomes that they do. Given the special circumstances surrounding the AIDS epidemic, reliance on the sets of variables identified during the pursuit of the evaluation of classical health evaluations is almost certainly shortsighted. Given that the AIDS evaluation literature is still in a formative stage, the use of inductive, qualitative interviews to identify respondent-centered perspectives on the consequences of an intervention is almost certainly necessary. The use of qualitative data collection efforts within larger evaluation efforts will avoid unnecessary limitations of identified correlates of change that will be imposed by the strict restriction of research to deductive designs. To restrict the identification of variables known to effect change in combination with interventions works to restrict the creation of innovative and cost-effective AIDS health policy options. Thus, the use of anthropological research methods—designed to identify respondent-identified reasons for intervention efficacy—can be directly used to improve intervention efficacy and expand intervention options.

Discussion

The research agenda outlined in this chapter has been defined to address the needs posed by the AIDS epidemic within a North American epicenter. The AIDS epidemic in San Francisco has not only resulted in a relentless nightmarish burden of morbidity and death but it may also strain local health care systems to the point of collapse. Given this extraordinary socio-medical crisis, the first priority in response to the epidemic must be prevention, the second, the care of those infected with HIV.

These are not priorities derived from the anthropological literature; rather, these priorities are derived from a public health understanding of the situation regarding the AIDS epidemic in San Francisco. Addressing the needs posed by the AIDS epidemic in this epicenter will require the combined expertise of representatives from a number of disciplines, including medicine, epidemiology, social work, biostatistics, nursing, health policy and economics, immunology, virology, neurology, as well as the medical/behavioral sciences (psychology, sociology, and anthropology). Since the nature of this epidemic requires a multidisciplinary public health response, priorities in the fight against AIDS have been defined across disciplines. Research projects that do not relate to these cross-disciplinary priorities do not hold great promise of being funded, understood, or used.

I argue in this chapter that the best use of anthropology in contributing to the fight against AIDS is to extend existent public health research agendas. The general neglect of anthropological research in extending public health agendas, particularly the lack of qualitative inductive research strategies, has diminished the effectiveness of public health and care efforts. Extending research agendas requires that anthropologists critically evaluate public health approaches to the epidemic and define how anthropological research strategies can make original contributions to existent public health efforts. Examples of such extensions include the need for exploratory, inductive studies of the conditions under which individuals take risks for HIV transmission and the inductive study of the conditions under which cost-effective and humane care for those suffering from HIV infection can be given.

This chapter describes findings from many different AIDS research projects. These studies would not have been possible without the willingness of research participants to devote time and energy in responding to very sensitive lifestyle questionnaires. This paper was supported by a National Institute of Mental Health/National Institute of Drug Abuse Center grant to the Center for AIDS Prevention Studies (MH42459) and a NIDA grant to develop a model of care for intravenous drug users with AIDS (DA 05673-02). Significant portions of this paper will also appear in a special monograph to be published by Congreso Internacional de Psicologia y Salud.

8

The Sociocultural Impacts of AIDS in Central and East Africa

DOUGLAS A. FELDMAN

The overall pattern of HIV transmission in central and East Africa is very different from the pattern found in North America and Europe. In central and East Africa, most HIV transmission, it is now known, occurs through heterosexual penile-vaginal intercourse (Piot et al. 1984; Van de Perre et al. 1984). The extent of HIV transmission through male homosexual activity in Africa has not yet been adequately researched, but certainly it is at most only a small but contributing factor to the overall rates of HIV seroprevalence (Feldman 1990a).

Recreational intravenous drug use is virtually unknown in Africa (Biggar 1986). The reuse of infected needles for medicinal purposes apparently plays a contributing role in HIV infection in some parts of central and East Africa (Mann et al. 1986) but less so in other parts of the region (Lepage et al. 1986). It is still uncertain if scarification and traditional curing practices currently play any role in HIV transmission (Good 1988).

HIV-infected pregnant mothers often infect their unborn children in Africa, as they do in North America and Europe. But with a considerably greater seroprevalence of HIV-infection among pregnant females in much of urban Africa, the problem of HIV-infected newborns is much larger there (Ryder et al. 1989). Breast-feeding most likely plays a small role in pediatric HIV transmission in Africa (Hira 1989).

HIV infection occurs very unevenly throughout Africa. It is at this point, mostly an urban disease (Haq 1988). One in four adult men and women under 50 in Lusaka, Zambia, are HIV-infected (Hira 1989). Even higher proportions of HIV-infected sexually active adult men and women have been found in the Rakai District of southwestern Uganda (Wawer 1988) and in Gulu and Lira in northern Uganda (Lwegaba 1988). While HIV-1 (Human Immunodeficiency Virus Type 1) continues to spread rapidly through much of urban central and East Africa, another AIDS-related retrovirus, HIV-2 (Human Immunodeficiency Virus Type 2) has begun spreading rapidly through the urban centers of West Africa from Senegal to Nigeria (Kanki et al. 1986). While a thorough comparison of the pattern of disease progression precipitated by these two retroviruses has yet to be made, it is now clear that HIV-2 does produce AIDS-like illness (Tumani et al. 1989). Projections estimate that about half of those who are HIV-1 infected with develop AIDS within ten years of seroconversion, and all or most will develop AIDS within a twenty-year period after seroconversion (Longini et al. 1989).

Many North Americans and Europeans believe that Africa is "doomed." After all, with no cure or effective vaccine in sight, there is nothing to stop the progression of the disease among the infected or the rate of seroconversions. The uninfected will become infected. The infected will become ill and die. The pandemic will spread from the African cities to the African countryside. And costly drug therapy, azidothymidine (AZT), and various experimental drugs, such as dideoxyinosine (ddI), will remain unavailable except perhaps to a small elite. Severe depopulation throughout Africa will occur, and the social fabric of daily life will disintegrate.

An alternative view often held by some Africans themselves is that the whole problem of AIDS in Africa has been greatly exaggerated. The problems of malnutrition, poverty, diarrheal disease (especially in children), and diseases for which cures exist but are simply not available far outweigh the impact of AIDS at this time. When we consider the spectrum of social and health ills that many Africans face constantly (unemployment, illiteracy, warfare, and the general scarcity of resources), AIDS is a relatively minor concern. Indeed, it is disarming that so much attention has been drawn by the West to AIDS in Africa when other health-related problems have for so long weighed more heavily and continue to go largely unnoticed. Clearly, in the West hunger and poverty are perceived as personally less threatening, at least among the middleclass, than AIDS.

Merritt (1989) has calculated that even the worst-case scenario with the spread of AIDS across Africa would only reduce the rate of population growth from about 3.5 percent per year to about 1.5 percent per year. Furthermore, there may be reason to believe that unknown factors may inhibit the spread of HIV infection in at least some rural areas of Africa. In one rural area of northern Zaire, the seroprevalence of HIV-1 did not increase above its prior 0.8 percent level after a decade (Nzilambi et al. 1988). Those advocating the optimistic view that the impact on AIDS upon Africa will not be disastrous might also argue that the resiliency of the extended family in Africa provides a strong social network for supporting family members with AIDS (Merritt, Lyerly, and Thomas 1988).

The truth probably lies somewhere between these two divergent views. Rather than talking about the social *impact* of AIDS in Africa, we must talk about the social *impacts* of AIDS in Africa. It is equally important to differentiate between the current impacts and those projected for five, ten, twenty years from now.

AIDS, unlike most other diseases, which strike primarily the very young or the old, attacks persons mainly in their twenties, thirties, and forties. In Africa, the typical person with AIDS is in his most economically productive years and is usually financially supporting or caring for a growing family. Children are left fatherless, motherless, or entirely orphaned. The family of the person with AIDS must endure not only the economic deprivation of the loss of a breadwinner or caretaker but also the psychological impact of caring for a chronically ill patient who is physically deteriorating before his loved ones (Ankrah 1988). AIDS is a socially stigmatizing disease that fosters feelings of fear, shame, guilt, and denial.

In Uganda, and perhaps elsewhere in Africa, if the wife develops AIDS-related symptoms before her husband does, even if she became infected from him and has been completely faithful to only him, the husband assumes that she has been unfaithful and casts her out of the household. In one rather poignant case in Masaka, Uganda, a woman who developed AIDS was immediately cast out of her home by her husband and was not allowed into her parents' home since through her presumed infidelity she had brought disgrace to her family. She stayed in a small hut not far from her home, ignored by all family members. As she progressively became more ill, her mother came to the hut to care for her. After a while, she died alone in the hut.

But when the husband in Uganda develops AIDS before the wife, it is her responsibility to take care of him. Often he is not able to continue working, and the family faces severe economic hardship. If the children become ill, further pressure is placed upon the burdened family. And if the wife falls ill to AIDS, she must take care of herself. When both parents die from AIDS, the orphaned children move in with the paternal grandparents. In the Rakai District, where one out of two adults is HIV-infected, the number of orphaned children has grown so rapidly and so pervasively that they are putting enormous stress on the extended family (Wawer 1988). Grandparents in Uganda rely on the structure of the extended family to give them emotional and financial support in their later years. With their sons and daughters-in-law gone, they are now responsible for the daily care and support of their grandchildren, some of whom may also be ill with AIDS. The grandparents increasingly are finding themselves straining to cope with this crisis. Should two sons and their wives die, leaving many newly orphaned children (some gravely ill), the grandparents are often unable to cope with this dilemma. The Ugandan government is now discussing the need to create state-run orphanages for the children of parents who had died of AIDS.

AIDS in Africa is found in all socioeconomic groups. In some areas of Africa AIDS seems to affect the poor as much as the middleclass and the wealthy. In other areas, such as Rwanda, the disease has affected the elite and middleclass disproportionately more (Torrey, Way, and Rowe 1988). As segments of the political and economic leadership of many African nations become ill or die, substantial stress may be put on national governments and economies.

HIV is a deceptively slow retrovirus. Even if there would be no more seroconversions among adults in urban Africa, which could not occur unless safer sex practices become universal and all needles are properly disinfected (two highly unlikely events at this time), one out of eight adults under fifty will be dead or chronically ill from AIDS within a decade in cities where one of four adults under fifty are HIV-seropositive. This is in addition to current morbidity and mortality rates among this cohort. There is no question that this will severely affect every segment of social life in urban Africa. Throughout much of urban central and East Africa, already overburdened hospitals and health clinics are facing increasing numbers of patients with AIDS or HIV-related disease. This pattern will continue to worsen. Recently, one physician in Lusaka, Zambia, called for the urgent construction of a second morgue in that city's main hospital (Bayley 1989).

For economic and other reasons, there has been considerable denial by both African governments and individuals of the catastrophic AIDS crisis. The case of Haiti may be instructive. Beginning in 1983, Haiti experienced a decline in tourism and foreign economic investment as a result of AIDS-related fear. Haitian-Americans were fired from their jobs in the United States because they were born in Haiti or had parents born there (Farmer 1990). It is possible that the ouster of "Baby Doc" Duvalier may have, at least in part, been caused by the further economic deterioration in Haiti from this decline in tourism and foreign economic investment. If true, then AIDS has directly toppled one government, and the fears in the mid-1980's of central and East African governments that such an event could occur in Africa as well were not so farfetched, after all. However, some African governments did overreact in their attempts to distance themselves from their growing AIDS crisis. Researchers were denied permission to conduct research or to publish their results; African and European researchers were not permitted to collaborate with foreign researchers on AIDS projects; at least two European physicians were expelled from two African countries either for giving too much information about AIDS to the press or for having said the wrong thing; one film crew was physically attacked by the police and expelled from a country; and reporters were denied access to information. The area that causes the greatest discomfort is, of course, the question of origins. Many feel that the allegations of an African origin of HIV-1 implicitly place blame upon all Africans. AIDS further stigmatizes already generally misunderstood or disliked populations. To date, the place of origin of HIV-1 remains unknown (Feldman 1990b). What is most peculiar is not why HIV-1 and HIV-2 emerged and spread but why so many other viruses have not. There is a veritable jungle of pathogenic human and animal viruses in the biosphere. With the advent of international jet travel, it is puzzling that there are not a dozen or more lethal AIDS-like diseases spreading relentlessly and unabated throughout the world. For that matter, given the growing number of biological warfare laboratories in nearly a dozen nations, it is surprising that laboratory accidents have not resulted in numerous synthetic pathogenic viruses being unleashed globally on unwary publics.

Today there seems to be less concern with the question of origins, and several African governments, following the prompting of the World Health Organization, have become more open to AIDS-related research, interventions, and discussions in the media and in public settings. Other governments are more reluctant to change. However, the fear of social stigma, loss of tourism, and decline of economic investment directly attributable to AIDS apparently has failed to materialize. Tourism in East Africa, for example, had been expanding recently. The general public loses most when a cloak of secrecy is maintained about AIDS in an African nation. AIDS is a preventable disease, and had there been widespread knowledge of safer sex practices and the risk reduction workshops necessary to effectuate the requisite change throughout central and East Africa a few years ago, there would undoubtedly be fewer persons HIV-infected today.

But what could have been is mostly beside the point. African governments need to move forward in developing AIDS education programs, including safer sex workshops. These must be culturally sensitive to the sexual mores, values, and actual practices for each culture. What is appropriate for the Bemba of northern Zambia is not appropriate for the Ila of south central Zambia. What is correct for the Karamajong of eastern Uganda is not correct for the Baganda of Kampala. The current practice of developing national AIDS education campaigns needs to be modified so that the information provided is more culture-specific. The values, attitudes, beliefs, and sexual practices of central and East Africa are diverse, complex, and heterogeneous. If the education campaign attempts to homogenize the sexual and social behavior throughout Africa so that the most restrictive are not offended, it is likely to subterfuge the rich and varied heritage of that continent. It is important to respect the diversity, including sexual diversity and sexual freedom, in all cultures and not to permit fear of AIDS to impose a universal morality of heterosexual monogamy and fidelity upon Africa, except in those locales where such practices have traditionally been highly valued. Safer sex in one culture may mean mutual fidelity and monogamy, but in another culture it may mean having many sexual partners while using condoms or non-penetrative sex practices.

Ngugi et al. (1988) in Nairobi have successfully demonstrated that AIDS risk-reduction programs do work in Africa. Female prostitutes who have gone through their program are frequently using condoms with their clients. Even though most Nairobi female prostitutes are already HIV-seropositive, their increased condom use is probably inhibiting the rate of disease progression and thus prolonging their own lives. It is one thing to get female prostitutes to have their clients use condoms, but it is quite another to ask wives to persuade their husbands to use condoms. Women in Africa wield little power in condom-use decision-making. The woman is often viewed as the "carrier," even though HIV-seropositive men would be at least as likely to infect HIV-seronegative women as vice versa, and a wife or girlfriend who insists that condoms be used would be regarded with deep suspicion by the husband or boyfriend. Research into effective virucides and virucidal devices is urgently needed for women who are not in a position to demand that their husbands or boyfriends use condoms.

There is also an immediate need for more condoms in Africa.

It has been estimated that sexually active men in Africa would need about 90 condoms per year (Kangas, Harris, and Shelton 1989). There are not nearly enough condoms available in Africa today to have much of an impact in slowing the spread of AIDS. Billions of condoms are needed each year.

The social impacts of AIDS in Africa are many and varied. For most rural Africans, AIDS is currently not an issue. While more HIV seroprevalence research is needed in rural African communities, the evidence that exists clearly supports the view that, with a few notable exceptions, AIDS in Africa remains a decidedly urban disease. It is likely that this will eventually change since there are few truly isolated communities in Africa. People migrate from the village to the city and back again all the time, and virions (viral entities) certainly do not self-destruct at the city line. Social scientists need to look very closely at migration patterns throughout Africa to better understand the epidemiologic spread of HIV (Brokensha 1988). Gradually, as the virus spreads into the countryside, new social impacts will emerge. HIV-1 is rapidly evolving, and it is perhaps likely that it will become less lethal in the coming decade or two (if it is after all to continue surviving in humans). This too will create a different kind of impact, as the virus results in fewer fatalities but longer-term chronic illnesses.

We face ethical issues as we encounter the challenge of AIDS in Africa. While many drugs are used to treat the opportunistic infections and cancers of AIDS, AZT is the only drug so far fully approved by the U.S. Food and Drug Administration for the treatment of HIV itself—though ddI and other drugs are now being made available in the United States on a "compassionate-use" basis without necessarily being part of a clinical research study. Though AZT often may cause serious side effects in some patients, it usually prolongs life and improves the quality of life of persons with AIDS and HIV-related illness. The problem for Africa is that it costs thousands of dollars per patient per year. What is the West's responsibility to the health of Africans? With very scarce medical resources in Africa, how can the expenditure of such costly treatments be justified when funds are not available for even some of the least expensive treatments for other diseases? Even if a fund is set up by the West for the distribution of AZT among some persons with AIDS in Africa, who is to decide who receives it and who does not? What criteria would be used?

The question of drug trials raises other ethical concerns. Drug trials for AIDS treatment could be carried out more economically and with larger sample sizes in areas of Africa where HIV seroprevalence is high. But should impoverished Africans be easily exploited subjects for experimentation? On the other hand, if the drugs were to be provided free by pharmaceutical companies and should prove effective, Africans could have much to gain from participation in such studies.

The prospect of large-scale vaccine trials, which will probably begin in Africa within the next few years, raises additional ethical issues. At the very least, it will be essential that participants understand the risks of a vaccine trial, the concept of experimentation, and the process of disease transmission. Their "consent forms" must be culture-specific. The role of the traditional healer is central to the health care of most Africans today, and it is vital that any national or local plan for AIDS control include an important role for traditional healers.

While this global pandemic has proven itself absolutely devastating from New York to Kinshasa, from Sao Paulo, Brazil, to Bujumbura, Burundi, from San Francisco to Bangkok, there may be some unintended benefits as a result of AIDS. The long-ignored medical and health needs of Africans are finally being noticed and taken seriously by some Western governments. Agencies such as AIDSTECH, AIDSCOM, WHO, U.S. AID, the British Medical Council, and others are beginning to spend tens of millions of dollars against AIDS in Africa. Disposable needles and syringes will not only slow the spread of HIV but will also be used to combat other diseases. Condoms will not only interfere with HIV transmission but will also curb runaway population growth and reduce the spread of other sexually transmitted diseases. Hospital equipment used for AIDS patients could also be used for other kinds of patients.

It is crucial that the serious challenge of AIDS in Africa be met head-on. The health and well-being of a continent is at stake. If Africans and their friends carefully plan for the health and medical needs of the continent as it faces the AIDS crisis, the most important step will have been taken in responding successfully to the challenge of AIDS in Africa.

Part of the data presented is derived from field trips to Rwanda (1985), Uganda (1988), and Zambia (1989). I would like to thank Dr. Ronald J. Prineas at the University of Miami School of Medicine for his comments on this paper.

9

Women, Children, and AIDS:
Research Suggestions

BETH E. SCHNEIDER

The early conceptualization of AIDS as a disease of gay men (presumed to be white) or of epidemiologically defined "risk groups" (IV drug users, Haitians, men having sex with men) foreclosed the recognition of the racial, class, and gender relations that frame the development of AIDS as a social problem and structure the social consequences of HIV infection. (See Schneider 1989 for a fuller discussion of the multiplicity of AIDS-related issues raised by the intersection of these three systems of inequality—race, class, and gender.) Early understandings of AIDS took for granted, with virtually no sustained analysis, that the vast majority of people with AIDS are men. The recognition of HIV-infection in women was, consequently, delayed. And while physicians observed infants and very young children with illnesses not unlike those of gay men as early as 1981 (Shilts 1988), their existence became most evident through the hostile response of fearful parents to children with AIDS in public schools throughout the country (Kirp 1989).

In the last three years, a change in direction among those concerned with AIDS has occurred, spurred in part by what is euphemistically dubbed in the press "the changing face of AIDS." While 90 percent of people with a diagnosed case of AIDS are male, women make up a small but increasing proportion of cases. Racial/ethnic minorities constitute 41 percent of the adult/adolescent cases of AIDS in the United States; 26 percent are blacks, 14 percent are Latinos (Centers for Disease

Control 1989b). Relative to the proportion of the total population, blacks and Latinos have an incidence of AIDS two or three times higher than whites for homosexual and bisexual males and over twenty times higher for heterosexual males. Half of the cases of AIDS among blacks and Latinos occurred among heterosexual IV drug users or their sexual partners. This high frequency of AIDS cases among racial/ethnic heterosexual IV drug users is responsible for the majority of the AIDS cases among black and Latin women and children (over 80 percent). Blacks and Latinos have greater relative risks of getting AIDS as IV drug users, bisexual men, heterosexual partners, and children than do whites (Selik, Castro, and Pappaioanou 1988).

When we think about women, children, and AIDS, and put them in the context of intersecting systems of race, class, and gender, a flood of complex research questions and policy dilemmas emerges. Race, class, and gender relations influence the experiences of people with AIDS, community and political reactions, the nature of institutional practice, and the dynamics of change in the society. More specifically, race, class, and gender are the three factors most determinant of people's health status and their degree of well-being. In concert, they will affect perceptions of health and illness, kinds and availability of care, modes of delivery, anticipated illnesses, and discourse and interaction patterns of doctor-patient relationships.

My discussion on HIV-infected women and children utilizes whatever is known from any source, often relying on reports from physicians and scholarship from psychologists, social workers, physicians, and historians and when necessary working from suggestive but often unsystematic evidence from the popular and alternative news media. With regard to women and children, I attempt to provide some sense of those issues, situational contexts, institutional spheres, and policy domains that beg for social scientific and sociological investigation.

HIV-Infected Women

Women constitute a small but continually increasing proportion of AIDS cases in the United States. Without attention to the intersection of gender, class, and race (Collins 1986), it is next to impossible to understand the particular situation of the vast majority of HIV-infected women. Women with AIDS do not fit into the AIDS profiles of gay males or IV drug-using males since neither of these adequately addresses some of the central physiological or sociopolitical differences between women and men and neither situates these women in their own unique historical and material conditions that shape their lives.

Nationally, drug use accounts for 52 percent of the female AIDS cases (Centers for Disease Control 1989b). Though regional differences exist, the proportion of women getting AIDS from male sexual partners has steadily increased since 1982 (Shaw 1988). Seventy-one percent of the women with AIDS are black and Latino, and of the total, over half reside in the New York/New Jersey Metropolitan Area and in Florida. In New York City, AIDS is now the major cause of death in women aged 25-29.

HIV-infected women do not constitute a self-conscious, politically active local or national community. Given their demographic and social profile, most of the women currently at highest risk or with AIDS are least likely to have access to adequate medical care or health insurance. The public, to the extent that it has awareness of these women, might easily scapegoat intravenous drug users and poor women of color, just as women typically encounter victim-blaming in response to their pregnancies, abortions, and sexually transmitted diseases and to the practice of prostitution (Schneider 1988; Buckingham and Rehm 1987; Shaw and Paleo 1986; Brandt 1985).

In addition, the life conditions and social-psychological stresses for women differ markedly from those of most men, especially white gay men about whom most research concerning AIDS has been undertaken and for whom most services concerning AIDS were organized. And all social-psychological dimensions that have an impact on stress (coping strategies, role strain, life events, and social support) are theoretically constructed differently for racial/ethnic groups (Kaplan 1983). Even medically, the women with AIDS are different. HIV-infected women continue to be misdiagnosed. Just recently, and only in the name of newborns, have pregnant women become part of certain drug trials from which previously they had been excluded (*New York Times,* July 11, 1989, C2).

Five areas of sociological research need to be explored in order to help women with AIDS. First, research is needed on female IV drug users. The materials that exist are limited. Until this decade, women as IV drug users were disregarded since they did not fit the "typescripts" of the drug addict (Robins 1980). These women are often still invisible in the research on IVDUs and AIDS in those instances in which studies do not report sex differences (Des Jarlais and Friedman 1988; Friedman et al. 1987). The literature on heroin use and women (Worth and Rodriguez 1987; Rosenbaum 1981) suggests that the women are different from men in that they come later to drug use, enter the heroin culture through introduction by a man, have larger habits, may rely on prostitution to support their drug use, and have children for whom they are caring. Some, but not all, of these women experience a conflict between their efforts to attain heroin and their mothering (Moore and Devitt 1989; Rosenbaun 1981).

Studies of women using heroin are insufficient to grapple with some factors such as the impact of membership in gangs on women users (Moore and Devitt 1989) or of the use of methadone or crack on women's lives (Bowser 1988). We still need to know more about how women become involved in drug use, especially in racial/ethnic communities. Factors that lead to the use of needle sharing among young women are not clear.

A second and broader avenue of investigation lies in delineating the unique quality of these women's lives as they confront the impact of AIDS on the emotional, psychological, and social aspects of their mothering. In understanding women with AIDS it is crucial to recognize this issue of motherhood. Eighty percent of the children with AIDS acquired it through their mothers who have AIDS or are HIV-infected. And the possibility of pediatric AIDS does raise innumerable issues for women about transmission to potential children and the impact of pregnancy on their own health (Schneider 1988; National Academy of Sciences 1986b).

Women at some risk for HIV infection have been urged to

postpone pregnancy until researchers learn more about a great number of medical quandaries. But a decision to forgo or terminate a pregnancy is typically not made lightly by most women. Women, whatever their cultural and religious heritage, confront issues in the AIDS epidemic about control over their reproductive futures and sexual desires, the meaning of children for them, values concerning abortion, and the inevitable confrontation with the biological clock. The distributions of unplanned pregnancies and sexually transmitted diseases parallel one another, revealing a highly structured sexual stratification in the society (Cates 1984; Darrow 1977). These issues have varying significance and impact among women of different class and racial backgrounds.

More specifically, black teenagers are more sexually active, are less likely to use contraception and abortion, and have a higher proportion of births to single women than whites (National Center for Health Statistics 1982; Zelnick and Kantner 1980). In part, these facts reflect historically different views of the value of children and black community support of single motherhood (O'Connell 1980; Thompson 1980), as well as the interlocking structures of race and class oppression. In addition, it is through motherhood that most Latinos affirm their status as women (Andrade 1982), though the meaning of mothering appears to vary depending on class position and gang membership (Moore and Devitt 1989). The limited research on female heroine users (mostly black) reveals that their motherhood is their singular claim to worthiness (Rosenbaum 1981).

Any understanding of motherhood in these women's lives must touch on the choices available to them within opportunity structures, their material conditions, and their perceptions of the possibilities for themselves and their children. For example, in a study that examined the decisions of HIV-positive and HIV-negative IV drug-using women as to whether to terminate pregnancies when informed of their status prior to twenty-four weeks' gestation, half of the positives and 44 percent of the negatives chose to terminate. For the positives, risk of perinatal transmission was an important concern, but the decisions to terminate were also related to other factors, such as prior elective abortion, negative emotional reaction to pregnancy, and whether the pregnancy was unplanned (Selwyn et al. 1989). Little is known from sociological research, though there are certainly hints from the media and social work and medical journals, about the impact the introduction of AIDS has for their lives. Some of the losses and changes are similar to those of gay men. But as mothers and as women of color, their relationship to their children and wider kin system is a different issue. HIV-infected women's activities as primary parents are utterly transformed. Family patterns may be disrupted (Drucker et al. 1988). Who will care for the mother and her children? What does care mean given the relative lack of resources? How does the kinship network help or hinder? How is a woman with AIDS able to care for her children? What does she feel about herself and her options? How does she decide what is best for her children when confronted with the fact that there are an estimated 50,000–100,000 children who are not sick but have been orphaned by AIDS (Lambert 1989b) and with a foster care system in major metropolitan areas that is already overtaxed and made more so by the unwillingness of foster families to take black children, fearing they may be AIDS-infected (Grossman 1988)?

A comparative study of racial and cultural variability in survival and support systems to adult women who are diagnosed with AIDS is needed to provide a detailed understanding of the ways in which they manage AIDS, the meanings women attribute to their illness or the illness of their children and the actions they take as a consequence. How have fictive and biological kin managed to care for one another in the face of fear, stigma, poverty, fragmented social relations, and racism? It is amazing that there is virtually no examination by sociologists of groups of mothers of PWAs (people with AIDS) or of the religious orders who take care of children with AIDS, that no one is systematically looking at how the kinship system of black women is working in dealing with AIDS or whether or not grandparents' strongly-felt rights and responsibilities to grand-children in Mexican-American families has lessened the impact of AIDS in poor and working-class families (Andrade 1982).

Documentation of these patterns is important in showing significant social organization where little is assumed and in demonstrating the strengths and limits of families and communities, and in so doing it can make a contribution to policy initiatives focused on the development of local institutional support systems.

A third area for research addresses itself to women and prevention of AIDS. There is as yet little systematic evidence to indicate what troubles women encounter when they introduce condoms into a sexual situation or talk about changing sexual practice. The age groups most affected by AIDS are precisely those that, because of the introduction and widespread use of birth-control pills and other female-centered contraceptives, never had to negotiate male-centered contraception. Others have little experience with *any* contraception (Mays and Cochran 1988). Young men may have no experience with condoms, and they may be sex and drug experimenters. Accounts from women with AIDS or female partners of HIV-infected men do indicate that some have experienced violence by their partners when they tried to raise the issue of safe sex and the use of condoms (Patton 1985; Richardson 1988). This introduction of a change in sexual terms necessarily reveals the structured nature of gender in sexual relations (Schneider and Gould 1987, 125). Much of the prevention material urges women to be even more responsible for sex than they were in the past, locating women as controllers of men's sexuality. Gender is revealed at every turn; for example, two of the four recent books about AIDS expressly for women base their arguments on the belief that men are not to be trusted in sexual matters (Kaplan 1987; Norwood 1987).

A number of researchable issues demand systematic cross-cultural exploration: How do women assess their risk, given the inconsistent reports about heterosexual transmission (Masters, Johnson, and Kolodny 1988; Gould 1988; Edwards 1987; Leisham 1987)? How are sexual partners chosen by single heterosexually active women and what kinds of sexual partners are chosen? In what ways is safer sex negotiated and how do heterosexual women speak about sex, given the sturdy cultural taboo against it (Webster 1984; Laws and Schwartz 1977)? How does cultural difference influence the response to prevention education (Mays and Cochran 1988)?

A fourth set of questions concerns the mobilization that has occurred in many racial/ethnic communities. When we talk about mobilization around AIDS, the demand on services, and challenges to entrenched systems, we are exploring the ways in which those who are underrepresented or invisible in government put forward a political agenda under less than ideal ideological and economic conditions (Altman 1987; Shilts 1988) in which systematic dismantling of the social programs and community action projects of the previous two decades had been occurring.

Questions about mobilization must also face up to the purported resistance of some leaders of racial/ethnic groups to acknowledge AIDS. We are just beginning to see some materials published by social scientists that explore systematically, rather than anecdotally, this resistance or the institutional response to AIDS that has emerged within these communities (Friedman et al. 1988; Greaves 1987). What actually were the sources of these leaders' resistance to dealing with AIDS? Answers to this question certainly would assist any understanding of the situation of women and children living with HIV-infection. How much of the conjecture and commentary by insiders and outsiders alike is accurate? Did homophobia, the stigma of the disease, the fear of ostracism, and increased direct racial assaults impede community leaders (Lee 1989)? Were early twentieth-century racial myths holding blacks responsible for syphilis (Fee 1988; Hammonds 1987) barriers to action? Was fear of deportation a hindrance for Mexican-Americans? Were the sources of resistance similar in Latin and black communities? Is it the case that Latin community members were more willing to talk about drugs than sex, African-American communities more willing to talk about sex than drugs?

As Shaw (1988) documents in her analysis of community organizing efforts around AIDS, the course of mobilization for women and racial/ethnic communities necessarily differs from that of the gay community given aggregate differences in wealth, political power, and positions in local government—that is, given significant differences in the ability to marshall resources. One of the most challenging but perhaps most fruitful ways to note the differences as well as to understand racial dynamics in the AIDS crisis is to study the processes through which the large urban AIDS organizations that were developed and sustained by resources and volunteers generated primarily by gay men confront the changing demographics of AIDS patients. What has been the history thus far of competition and accommodation? Have new social movement organizations emerged as a result of entrenchment or encouragement of these larger groups?

What resources and institutions have been used by particular communities to respond to HIV? In the mobilization that has occurred, how significant has been the role of the traditionally active leaders and institutions, such as churches, in black and the various Latin communities? Some social history analysis on the Catholic church in one large metropolitan area indicated considerable efforts to provide compassionate care but minimal effort to offer or support prevention education (Horrigan 1988). Many more analyses of other institutions and over longer periods of time are needed. Has the impetus for action come from new groups within the community or, as some have noted (Johnson, Munoz, and Pares 1988), from traditionally silent persons, such as racial/ethnic gay men? Who is speaking for HIV-infected women? What organized responses have there been from the women themselves, from feminist organizations, from racial/ethnic community organizations?

A fifth area of research focuses on policy. Analyses are needed of the state's response to demands from people with AIDS and how those demands have changed over time as the medical situation alters and the demographics of the new cases change. The state may mobilize resources; it may also initiate repression. State apparatus at various governmental levels organizes policies through enforcement of discrimination law, control of education, and procedures to detain and punish. How have women and children with HIV-infection been affected by social welfare and public health policy both regarding AIDS and concerning other matters that have indirect impact on their lives?

For women, AIDS threatens further to legally and medically dictate the processes of pregnancy and childbirth (Rothman 1987; Zimmerman 1987). Women are in a particularly critical situation in this regard as the implications of some policy proposals force them to confront ethical and rights issues unique to women. The combination of new reproductive surveillance technologies, discussions of fetal rights, and the posing of women's rights against the rights of the fetus are all made manifest in discussions of both AIDS and drug epidemics. Renewed attention is called to women's rights concerning sex and reproduction—women's rights to control sexual practice, women's rights to privacy, women's rights to sexual and other freedoms, women's rights to be pregnant (Terry 1989; Murphy 1988).

Recent Supreme Court and lower court decisions have a bearing on the kinds of ethical dilemmas and practical choices women will face. Access to abortion and prenatal care are class issues; freedom of choice without economic means to avail oneself of that choice is meaningless. The poor have had the fewest opportunities to exercise control over reproductive activities. The recent practice of incarcerating drug-using pregnant women serves to exaggerate further the problems for select groups of women. In California and elsewhere, state funding has been cut for family planning clinics, resulting in no birth control, no medical examinations, no treatment for sexually transmitted diseases, and no tests for HIV for working poor and unemployed persons (Scott 1989). In New York City, HIV-infected women are being denied abortions in non-hospital settings, despite various city and state laws prohibiting providers from refusing to treat people who are infected (Taravella 1989). Policies such as these contradict some of the best efforts of public health professionals.

The ethical issues point to research questions for social scientists. How have the communities in which HIV-infected women primarily reside responded to public messages to curtail sexual activity or forgo childbearing? How do women vary in their response to a possible threat of mandatory abortions for infected pregnant women? What is the decision-making calculus women use or will use to weigh these often competing rights? What political struggles might ensue among organized groups already concerned with issues such as sex education or abortion and family planning, and how will their outcomes affect HIV-infected women?

Children with HIV-Infection

In considerations of HIV-infection in children, there are typically two sorts of portraits: the first, an infant, usually African-American, abandoned to a hospital, born to an IV drug-using mother (Grossman 1988; Heagarty 1987); the second, a ten-year-old white child with HIV-infection from blood products who is refused entry into school because of the objections of parents in the local community (Kirp 1989). These powerful images conveyed by the media constitute the beginnings of relatively accurate portrayals of the experience of children with AIDS in the United States.

While the images are powerful, the experience of HIV-infected children has not been very intensively studied by social scientists. With a few exceptions, most of what we know has come from the experience of social workers and physicians and has been discussed in the National Academy of Sciences books (1986a, 1986b) and the recent Presidential Commission Report on HIV (1988). A brief summary of what is known about these children suggests some directions fro research in the next decade.

According to the Presidential Commission on HIV, by 1991 there will be approximately 10,000–20,000 diagnosed cases of AIDS in children in the United States. Currently, most cases of AIDS in children (80 percent) are a result of perinatal transmission from infected mothers; 11 percent of the children with HIV infection acquired the virus from transfusions, and 6 percent are hemophiliacs (Centers for Disease control 1989b). The vast majority of the children who acquired the disease perinatally suffer the multiple impacts of racial and class oppression in the form of inadequate health care and support services to which their mothers are also subjected. Moreover, those children not infected perinatally suffer from the responses of others—the persistent fear of contagion and the expressions of homophobia.

The factors in perinatal transmission and efforts at early

diagnosis have been and continue to be extensively studied by medical practitioners (National Academy of Sciences 1986a). At present, there is considerable understanding of the kinds of infections and illnesses children suffer and the means necessary to treat them. Because HIV infection in an asymptomatic newborn may not be diagnosed accurately for ten to eighteen months, all seropositive infants require monitoring for this length of time.

Whatever the mode of transmission, the children share similar infections. Clinical trials of AZT are now occurring for children living with AIDS, but overall, experimental trials for pediatric patients lag far behind those for adults. Children's economic situations do have a significant impact on the course of their illness. Like their parents, many of the children who rely on public hospitals, which do not dispense experimental medications, are missing out on the opportunity to forestall the course of disease (Lambert 1989c).

The children infected through transfusion or blood products tend to live longer than the infants infected perinatally. They suffer the effects of having their once ordinary lives altered significantly by discrimination, isolation, or the sense of abandonment they feel if relationships with friends and peers at school change (Kirp 1989; Presidential Commission on HIV 1988). Unlike the babies, these children have to face directly many of the same issues as adults living with AIDS, such as the need to confront stigma and death. Surprisingly, there does not seem to be a sociologist or developmental psychologist attempting to understand the experience of these children, many of whom have entered or soon will enter adolescence.

As suggested in the earlier discussion on women living with AIDS, a special problem of many children with HIV infection is the unavailability of one or both parents because of AIDS and/or drug addiction, necessitating long-term or permanent hospitalization in the absence of any other available care setting (Heagarty 1987). Infected mothers and newborns are frequently from poor, drug-using families that rely on Medicaid and on the care provided by public hospitals (Drucker et al. 1988; Shaw and Paleo 1986). HIV-infected infants born to mothers who may be unable or unwilling to care for them occasionally are left in hospital wards. Drug-addicted seropositive babies are also often low weight and born to mothers who had no prenatal care, requiring prolonged hospital stays and possibly needing neo-natal intensive care. But these children are beginning life under dire conditions even when their mothers are themselves healthy and available to provide care.

Most of the perinatal transmission cases die of HIV-related complications before the age of three, though a few children have lived as long as ten years. In areas with high pediatric HIV infection, special pediatric units have been developed to serve the children. Children remain in these units even when they no longer need hospital attention. It is quite usual to find that when children are discussed by government officials and medical economists, it is the cost of their care that is most highlighted. Not that these costs are insignificant: it costs ap-proximately $1,200 per day for hospital care compared to $100 per day for specialized foster care (Presidential Commission Report on HIV 1988). While the care offered takes into account their medical, social, and educational needs, the setting is not conducive for any child's long-term growth. Again, child devel-opment specialists need to explore short- and long-term social and psychological responses and consequences.

Despite the unavailability of foster care, some HIV-infected children have been taken in or adopted by orphanages and foster parents, often single heterosexuals or gay and lesbian adults. Though the numbers are currently small, longitudinal studies of the emotional, medical, and intellectual impact of these home contexts on parent surrogates and, of course, on the children would fill gaps in a picture of care that has focused primarily on the hospital setting.

There are other children affected by AIDS. Some legal schol-ars have noted that children who are relatives of HIV-infected persons but who are themselves unaffected medically need pro-tections from discrimination and exclusion under section 504 of the Rehabilitation Act of 1973 and the equal protection clause of the Constitution (MacFarlane 1989). Drucker et al. (1988) raise additional issues concerning children's efforts to deal with the uncertainty of a parent's death, the loss of a residence, and the fear for their own health. Many more such systematic social science efforts to study pediatric AIDS and these children are obviously needed.

The experience of HIV-infected children perhaps best highlights the gap between the need for treatment and services and the level of provision. This gap is familiar to all who are concerned with social welfare, drug use, or urban politics. AIDS simply adds to the emergency and highlights the lack of services. Among the problems in services confronted by HIV-infected children and those who care for them are an overburdened and underfinanced foster care system, a lack of Medicaid coverage for home or community-based health care, a lack of supportive services to nuclear and extended families, and few group homes (Drucker et al. 1988; Presidential Commission on HIV 1988; Grossman 1988). Since the problem of HIV-infected children continues to increase and since these particular children have no support systems, resources, or political lobbyists separate from the families and communities of which they are members, policy analysts should now attend to who will become the allies of children with AIDS and under what conditions.

Most cases that emerge in the future will be instances of perinatal transmission rather than through blood or blood products. And the problem is quite extraordinary. For example, initial results of the ongoing New York State serosurvey of all newborns (200,000 a year) have shown 2.4 percent of all births in the Bronx to be positive for HIV antibodies, the highest level in the state; where drug use is widespread, the rates are even higher. Also an anonymous serosurvey conducted among abortion patients at a South Bronx clinic found 6.7 percent of those patients over 25 years old to be positive. Drucker and Vermund (1989) recently reported that these figures, coupled with some for emergency room studies, indicate an advanced state of infection, with seroprevalence patterns similar to those in some central Africa areas and with "ominous implications" for children, especially newborns in the area. In addition, the growing problem of HIV infection among adolescents requires systematic efforts in the research on drug initiation practices for a number of drugs and the scope of education to new users.

Kirp's (1989) study offers a serious effort to explore systematically the community dynamics surrounding attendance of

HIV-infected children in public schools. Most of his cases occurred at a particular historical period in which public panic and mistrust of health officials was high (Shilts 1988; Altman 1987). Recently, the National Association of State Boards of Education (1989) has issued guidelines emphasizing confidentiality in the handling of future cases. Hence, in addition to the kinds of research proposed on the life trajectory of the perinatally-infected and their social support system, social history analyses continue to be needed on current and future reactions to the increasing number of children who will survive to go to school.

Conclusion

The social science research on women and children with HIV-infection is relatively new; social scientists are still relying on the work of other professionals to understand the complex social relationships of women and children to HIV-infection. A research agenda for these groups in the near future must invariably grapple with their social location and the unique problems posed by multiple oppression, as well as their relative powerlessness within social and political structures. Research that takes special care to deal with the particular subjectivity of these persons, to see the problem of AIDS from their point of view, is desperately needed to deal with a rapidly growing medical problem and to deal respectfully with ongoing and potential devastation to both kin and community.

10

Federal Funding in AIDS Activity

ERNESTINE VANDERVEEN

The U.S. Public Health Service (PHS) is organizationally a part of the Department of Health and Human Services and is the principal health agency in the federal government. In the past decade, the PHS has been widely criticized for inadequate and untimely response to the AIDS epidemic. The purpose of this discussion is not to defend, refute, substantiate, or amplify these charges, but to attempt a systematic look at trends in the expenditure of fiscal resources by the federal government on AIDS-related activities. While the focus of this discussion is on research, I would suggest that AIDS expenditures are not easily triaged nor precisely calculated for a variety of reasons. Nevertheless, financial data analyses and published reports on AIDS-associated quantifiable costs are becoming available (Winkenwerder, Kessler, and Stolec 1989: Intergovernmental AIDS Reports 1989).

In the early years of the epidemic, few people knew or cared much about AIDS. The few clinicians and researchers who struggled with understanding AIDS were largely isolated in their clinical settings and laboratories. The discovery of the disease-causing virus and the routes of transmission were hailed as major breakthroughs in the popular and scientific media, and the most intimate of personal behaviors became the focus of attention in our national anxiety about how to stop the spread of the disease-causing Human Immunodeficiency Virus (HIV).

Also in the early 1980s, the Reagan administration greatly feared the advancement of a "liberal agenda" that they perceived would become a reality through research on human development and social structures. "Social Engineering" was the term used to describe adverse consequences such scientific activity would bring about. Applications for support for socially contaminated studies were returned by the grant-awarding agencies without action and, of course, without money. Research on sexual behavior was particularly hard-hit. As behavioral and social science research became less fundable, researchers, administrators, and department chairs had to reorient scientific programs toward the more respectable (and fundable) hard sciences. Long-standing disputes about the value and legitimacy of behavioral and social science research were re-ignited and continue to blaze, in spite of abundant advice on the critical and urgent need for such research. Today a major void exists in what is known about human behaviors most frequently involved in transmitting the HIV. Because of chronic inadequate funding, we still know little about almost all health-compromising sexual behaviors. We know much less about ways to change those behaviors; our knowledge base in this area remains rudimentary (National Academy of Sciences, 1986a, 230-31; 1989).

Against this backdrop, the voice and image of the surgeon general became known and was widely heard even if not heeded. Many conferences were held, commissions established, and experts appointed to various bodies to study the problem and tell the nation what to do. Much advice remains unheeded, and, in keeping with the cure-orientation of modern medicine, the search for magical technology continues at ever-higher cost. Little change is noted in the general trend and direction of health-related research.

The question of who pays and how the costs are borne becomes increasingly important as the numbers of HIV-infected persons and diagnosed AIDS cases continue to grow. The federal government has allocated increasing amounts of money primarily to research, as shown in table 10.1, which is based on information published by Winkenwerder, Kessler, and Stolec (1989) and depicts summarized federal spending from 1982 through 1989 by department. The Department of Health and

Human Services (DHHS) expenditures account for nearly 90 percent of all funds for AIDS expended to date. A number of other federal departments and agencies are also engaged in AIDS research, treatment, prevention, and education, most notably the Department of Veterans Affairs and the Department of Defense.

When looking at spending by functional activity, as shown in table 10.2, it is apparent that twice as much has gone for research ($2.2 billion) as has been spent in prevention ($1.1 billion). Medical care spending, primarily through entitlement programs, accounts for $1.9 billion, while cash-assistance payments to disabled patients with AIDS is relatively small—$0.3 billion. As the epidemic progresses and more infected persons become ill, this figure is likely to increase.

Half of the cumulative AIDS-designated PHS funds are spent by the National Institute of Health (NIH), $1.6 billion primarily for investigation into the pathogenesis and clinical manifestations of HIV infection and the research and development of anti-HIV drugs. The Centers for Disease Control (CDC) is the agency primarily responsible for HIV and AIDS case surveillance activity, epidemiological studies, analysis and reporting of trend data, public information and education, and prevention, including HIV testing and counseling. Through 1989, the CDC share of cumulative PHS funds was 30 percent ($938 million). The Alcohol, Drug Abuse and Mental Health Administration (ADAMHA) share totals 11 percent ($352 million) and supports research in behavioral, biological, and drug abuse aspects of HIV transmission and infection, as well as research in clinical manifestations of AIDS with relevance to drug use and central nervous system sequelae.

The Health Resources and Services Administration (HRSA) supports programs relating to delivery of patient care and services, including demonstrations and education projects. The Food and Drug Administration (FDA) has responsibility for evaluating and approving all new drugs, vaccines, and HIV diagnostic tests; regulating blood banks; monitoring the safety of the nation's blood supply; and ensuring effectiveness of condoms and rubber gloves.

Other offices and agencies such as the Office of Minority

Table 10.1. Federal Spending for AIDS According to Department (Millions of dollars[a])

	1982	1983	1984	1985	1986	1987	1988	1989	Total
Health/human Services:									
PHS									
NIH	3	22	44	64	135	261	468	604	1,600
CDC	2	6	14	33	62	136	305	379	938
ADAMHA	0	1	3	3	12	48	112	174	352
HRSA	0	0	0	0	15	42	37	55	149
FDA	0	0	1	9	10	16	30	63	129
Other PHS	0	0	0	0	0	0	4	14	19
HCFA	0	10	30	75	140	215	360	546	1,376
SSA	0	0	6	13	33	51	88	138	329
Other	0	0	0	0	0	0	3	6	9
Veterans Affairs	0	5	6	10	23	54	83	144	325
Defense	0	0	0	0	79	74	52	67	272
Other Depts.	0	0	0	0	1	2	5	4	12
TOTAL	6	44	104	207	509	899	1,548	2,195	5,511

[a]Dollar amounts are rounded to nearest million. Because of rounding, columns may not add to totals shown. Source: Winkenwerder et al. 1989.

Health and the Indian Health Service also have various coordinating and education activities. It must be noted that while federal research funding is provided primarily by the PHS agencies, the Department of Defense (DOD) and the Department of Veterans Affairs (DVA) also fund basic and clinical research. However, principal activities of these department are in HIV testing in the case of the DOD and in providing medical care for veterans with AIDS in the DVA health care system. (The VA system continues to report approximately two hundred new AIDS cases per month, and they are increasingly being reported from mid-America, according to the DVA program office.) In short, the federal effort in research is large and is expended primarily on basic biomedical studies.

What lies ahead, and what is the outlook for continued funding at this level? Acknowledging that some infectious diseases—measles for example—are still not eradicated even when

Table 10.2. Federal Spending for AIDS According to Activity (Millions of dollars[a])

	1982	1983	1984	1985	1986	1987	1988	1989	Total	%
Research										
PHS	3	22	57	83	164	317	607	815	2,067	
DOD	0	0	0	0	38	22	12	27	98	
DVA	0	0	2	3	3	6	8	14	34	
Other	0	0	0	0	0	1	1	1	2	
Subtotal	3	22	59	86	204	345	626	856	2,201	40
Education and prevention										
PHS	2	7	4	25	55	145	321	388	947	
DOD	0	0	0	0	18	25	26	26	94	
Other	0	0	0	0	0	2	8	37	47	
Subtotal	2	7	4	25	73	172	354	450	1,088	20
Medical care										
MEDICAID (federal share)[b]	0	10	30	70	130	200	330	490	1,260	
DVA	0	5	5	8	20	47	74	103	261	
PHS	0	0	0	0	16	41	29	87	173	
DOD	0	0	0	0	23	27	15	15	80	
MEDICARE[b]	0	0	0	5	10	15	30	55	115	
Other	0	0	0	0	1	1	1	2	4	
Subtotal	0	15	35	83	199	331	480	751	1,893	34
Cash assistance										
Disability ins.[b]	0	0	5	10	25	40	70	110	260	
Suppl. sec. ins.	0	0	1	3	8	11	18	28	69	
Subtotal	0	0	6	13	33	51	88	138	329	6
Grand total	6	44	104	207	509	899	1,548	2,195	5,511	100

[a]Dollar amounts are rounded to nearest million. Becasue of rounding, columns may not add to totals shown.   [b]Disability insurance: Estimates on these lines have been rounded to the nearest $5 million by actuaries at the Health Care Financing Administration of the Social Security Administration. Source: Winkenwerder et al. 1989.

technology-based prevention is available and that others—like tuberculosis, for which effective treatment is available—are still not eradicated, should the current research course continue to be supported with billions of dollars? There is increasing concern about the proportion of federal spending on AIDS research, education, and prevention relative to that spent for other diseases. Table 10.3 summarizes federal spending in fiscal year 1989 for six major diseases. The argument is made that diseases that account for many more deaths than AIDS are receiving insufficient portions of available fiscal resources ("Biomedical Dollars and Body Counts" 1989).

A number of arguments can be made in favor of continued large outlays for AIDS research, including uncertainties about the magnitude of the epidemic; the burden of death from AIDS on young people; the finding that the HIV is far more complex than once believed; the rationale that money spent on AIDS research advances science and contributes to the understanding of other diseases; and the international perspective that the U.S. has a responsibility to develop a cure or vaccine, as 5–10 million people, mostly in poor countries, are thought to be infected (Winkenwerder, Kessler, and Stolec 1989). There are many complex factors that influence the future level of spending for AIDS, though their impact is hard to predict:

1. If a treatment for preventing HIV infection from progressing to AIDS were found, care and social services costs would surely increase dramatically. It is likely that persons at risk would seek testing in greater numbers and early treatment would be sought by persons with positive results.

2. The spread of the virus could increase or decrease more rapidly than has been observed or predicted.

3. Changes in laws could occur to extend insurance and/or health care coverage.

4. Unanticipated budgetary and political pressures could influence appropriations.

5. Options not yet seriously considered, such as national reordering of research and health care priorities, could occur.

What appear to be viable options? And will those options be considered seriously in today's political environment? A first option is to begin to mainstream or integrate AIDS as just

Table 10.3. Federal Spending in Fiscal Year 1989 for Research on Education about and Prevention of Major Diseases

	Millions of dollars
Cancer[a]	1,449
AIDS and HIV	1,306
Heart disease	1,008
Diabetes	267
Stroke and hypertension	182
Alzheimer's disease	127

[a]Total National Cancer Institute appropriations for 1989, minus amount devoted to AIDS-related activities. This figure may underestimate the true total federal expenditure (complete data are not available). Source: Winkenwerder et al. 1989.

another infectious disease in our collective pool of diseases, one for which we do not yet have a cure or a treatment. Albeit we do know how it can be prevented, we simply do not know how to induce and sustain the appropriate behaviors on a scale large enough to curb the epidemic. Some benefits could be realized from converting AIDS to a respectable disease in the medical and ultimately the public perception. There may be positive implications for overcoming associated social stigma and discrimination. Some analogies can be made: in the area of addictions, alcoholism has become, if not a respected disease, at least not as stigmatized as addiction acquired through illicit drug use. Changes in public and medical perceptions might enable science to move forward in pursuit of useful research to general knowledge with wider application, particularly in sexually transmitted disease and drug abuse related disorders. The AIDS epidemic gives a valid medical rationale for drawing attention and resources to the devastating consequences of drug abuse. We have the potential to move drug abuse issues from the emotionally laden moral or criminal behavior arena to the public health domain, which in turn can lead to more effective treatment and interventions based on behavior change. Suffice it to say that nobody was interested in intravenous drug abusers until it was recognized that drug injection could become a major transmission vector (and that drug users are also sexually active). Today, the concern for the spread of HIV infection focuses primarily on drug use issues.

A second option is to reorder research priorities. The recent report from the Senate Committee on Appropriations quite clearly states that the ADAMHA research portfolio in social and behavioral sciences should be expanded and directs the agency to "research more aggressively the ramifications of the disease." It is of interest that in the House report on the same bill, H.R. 2990, separation of AIDS appropriations from regular institute budgets is not mentioned. This is for the purpose of permitting "scientific managers greater flexibility to allocate research dollars to the most promising areas of science" (U.S. Congress, 1990a, 89; 1990b, 176). It remains unclear what effect such flexibility will have on priorities for the social and behavioral sciences.

Third, and from a more global perspective, can we take what we have already learned from the AIDS experience and begin to work toward developing a health care system that can handle a crisis like AIDS? In the opinion of many both in and outside the health community who have assessed the AIDS phenomenon, the current state of affairs is not adequate to deal with diseases of the magnitude and complexity of AIDS and the other "killer diseases." We are learning that most diseases have social dimensions and that a disease can no longer be viewed as a biological, organic phenomenon requiring a single cure that ever-advancing technology promises to provide. Quite rapidly we are learning that the people who are the most vulnerable to HIV infection are also the most vulnerable to other diseases associated with neglect, poverty, homelessness, and all the other ills of disenfranchised individuals and groups. Has health care in the United States through real or artificial barriers become separated from the larger society? Growing numbers of Americans are said to have no access to health care, giving credence to this speculation.

And finally, can we turn the focus from cure to prevention for those diseases we know how to prevent? An example can be seen in the recognized association between drug abuse and the spread of the AIDS epidemic. A sizable and commendable effort is under way to develop medications for treatment of cocaine and other drug addictions (Waldrop 1989). In treatment approaches found to be useful for addicted persons, poor patient compliance with medication and treatment regimes remains a major problem. Patients are frequently unwilling to take even very effective medication, a common human behavior that hinders successful treatment of many disorders. Although treatment is successful for many addicted persons, the life problems most directly associated with addiction are frequently impossible to resolve. These problems in the real world of the patient begin all over again in the health-compromising environment of the drug abuse lifestyle in which none of the individual's basic human needs are likely to be met.

It is obvious that the advent of AIDS has served to complicate and multiply the many tasks that challenge the public health community. It may take a long time and much persuasion to turn current research trends in a direction that will enable development of a balanced knowledge base. Only an integrated and equal partnership among the biological, behavioral, and social sciences can accomplish such a goal. The behavioral and social aspects of health and disease present the scientific community with both opportunity and challenge.

The opinions expressed in this chapter are the views of the author and do not necessarily reflect the official position of the National Institute on Alcohol Abuse and Alcoholism or any other part of the U.S. Department of Health and Human Services.

References Cited

Abrams, E. 1990. Personal communication with E. Drucker regarding unpublished data, Harlem Hospital Center, New York City.

Agnos, A. 1988. Testimony of Mayor Art Agnos to the Presidential Commission on AIDS. San Francisco, Mar. 25. Quoted in *An Epidemic of Loss: AIDS in San Francisco's Gay Male Community, 1988-1993*, ed. R. Baker and J. Moulton. San Francisco: San Francisco AIDS Foundation.

Alderman, M. et al. 1988. "Predicting the Future of the AIDS Epidemic and Its Consequences for the Health Care System of New York City." *Bulletin of the New York Academy of Medicine* 64 (2): 175-83.

Alexander, P. 1988. *Prostitutes Prevent AIDS*. San Francisco: Prostitutes Education Project.

Altman, D. 1987. *AIDS in the Mind of America*. New York: Anchor.

Andrade, S. 1982. "Social Science Stereotypes of the Mexican-American Woman: Policy Implications for Research." *Hispanic Journal of Behavior Science* 4: 223-44.

Andre, L. 1987. "Le S.I.D.A. A-T-IL Deja Existe?" *Medicine Tropicale* 47, 4: 229-30.

Ankrah, E.M. 1988. Personal communication with D.A. Feldman.

Arno, P.S. 1986. "The Non-Profit Sectors Response to the AIDS Epidemic: Community-Based Services in San Francisco." *American Journal of Public Health* 76, 11: 1325-30.

——— et al. 1989. "Economic and Policy Implications of Early Intervention in HIV Disease." *Journal of the American Medical Association* 262, 11: 1493-98.

Aubry, P. 1989. "Le SIDA dans les Caribes en Oceanie: Editorial." *Medicine Tropicale* 49: 9-10.

Auerbach, D.M. et al. 1984. "Cluster of Cases of Acquired Immune Deficiency Syndrome: Patients Linked by Sexual Contact." *American Journal of Medicine* 76 (Mar.): 487-92.

AVOL 1987. Articles of Incorporation, 1-2.

Bachrach, C.F., and W. D. Mosher. 1984. "Use of Contraception in the United States, 1982." *Advance Data from Vital and Health Statistics* 102 (Dec. 4): 1-8.

Bailey, N. 1975. *The Mathematical Theory of Infectious Diseases.* London: Griffin.

Baker, R., and J. Moulton, eds. 1988. *An Epidemic of Loss: AIDS in San Francisco's Gay Male Community, 1988-1993.* San Francisco: San Francisco AIDS Foundation.

Barry, M., J. Mellors, and R. Bia. 1984. "Haiti and the AIDS Connection." *Journal of Chronic Diseases* 37: 592-95.

Bayley, A. 1989. "Home Care in a City." Paper presented at the Second National STD/AIDS Seminar. Lusaka, Zambia, Mar.

Becker, M.H., and J.G. Joseph. 1988. "AIDS and Behavioral Change to Reduce Risk: A Review." *American Journal of Public Health* 78, 4: 394-410.

Berry, B. 1972. "Hierarchical Diffusion: The Basis of Developmental Filtering and Spread in a System of Growth Centers." In *Growth Centers in Regional Economic Development,* ed. N. Hansen, 108-23. New York: Free Press.

Biegel Institute for Health Policy and the United Hospital Fund of New York. 1988. *New York City's Hospital Occupancy Crisis: Caring for a Patient Population.* New York: United Hospital Fund.

Biggar, R. 1986. "The AIDS Problem in Africa." *Lancet I: 79-83.*

———. 1987. "AIDS in Subsaharan Africa." *Cancer Detection and Prevention Supplement* 1: 487-91.

———, M. Melbye et al. 1985. "ELISA HTLV Retrovirus Antibody Reactivity Associated with Malaria and Immune Complexes in Healthy Africans." *Lancet* II: 520-23.

"Biomedical Dollars and Body Counts." 1989. *Science* 246, 1426: 34.

Bowser, B. 1988. "Crack and AIDS: An Ethnographic Impression." *MultiCultural Inquiry and Research on AIDS Quarterly Newsletter* 2, 2 (Spring): 1-2.

Brandt, A. 1985. *No Magic Bullet: A Social History of Venereal Disease in the United States since 1880.* London: Oxford Univ. Press.

Brokensha, D. 1988. "Overview: Social Factors in the Transmission and Control of AIDS." In *AIDS in Africa: The Social and Policy Impact,* ed. N. Miller and R.C. Rockwell, 167-74. Lewiston, N.Y.: Edwin Mellon.

Brookmeyer, R., and M. Gail. 1986. "Minimum Size of the Acquired Immunodeficiency Syndrome (AIDS) Epidemic in the United States." *Lancet* II (Dec.): 1320-22.

Brooks-Gunn, J., C. Boyer, and K. Hein. 1988. "Preventing HIV Infection and AIDS in Children and Adolescents." *American Psychologist* 43: 958-64.

Brown, L. 1981. *Innovation Diffusion: A New Perspective.* London: Methuen.

Brun-Vizinet, F. et al. 1984. "Prevalence of Antibodies to Lymphadenopathy-Associated Retrovirus in African Patients with AIDS." *Science* 226: 453-56.

Brundage, J.F. et al. 1989. "Spatial Diffusion of the Human Immunodeficiency Virus Infection Epidemic in the United States, 1985-87." *Annals of the Association of American Geographers* 79, 1 (Mar.): 25-43.

Brunet, J., E. Boubet, and J. Leibowitch. 1983. "Acquired Immunodeficiency Syndrome in France." *Lancet* I: 700-701.

Buckingham, S.L., and S. Rehm. 1987. "AIDS and Women at Risk." *Health and Social Work Journal* 12, 1 (Winter): 5-11.

Byers, R.H., Jr. et al. 1988. "Estimating AIDS Infection Rates in the San Francisco Cohort." *AIDS* 2 (June): 207-10.

Bygbjerg, I. 1983. "AIDS in a Danish Surgeon (Zaire, 1976)." *Lancet* I: 295.

Cabinet for Human Resources, Division of Epidemiology (Kentucky). 1989. Monthly Report: "AIDS in Kentucky."

Cabinet for Human Resources, Division of Epidemiology (Kentucky). 1990. Monthly Report: "AIDS in Kentucky.

Casetti, E. 1972. "Generating Models by the Expansion Method: Applications to Geographic Research." *Geographical Analysis* 4: 81-91.

———. 1982. "Mathematical Modeling and the Expansion Method." In *Statistics for Geographers and Social Scientists,* ed. R. Mandal. New Delhi, India: Concept.

———. 1986. "The Dual Expansion Method: An Application to Evaluating the Effects of Population Growth on Development." *IEEE Transactions of Systems, Man and Cybernetics* SMC-16: 29-39.

Castro, K. et al. 1988. "Transmission of HIV in Belle Glade, Florida: Lessons for Other Communities in the United States." *Science* 239: (Jan. 8) 193-97.

Catania, J.A., S.M. Kegeles, and T.J. Coates. 1990. "Towards an Understanding of Risk Behavior: The CAPS AIDS Risk Model (ARRM)." *Health Education Quarterly* 17:53-72.

Cates, W., Jr. 1984. "Sexually Transmitted Diseases and Family Planning." *Journal of Reproductive Medicine* 29, 5 (May): 317-22.

Centers for Disease Control. 1982. "Update on Acquired Immune Deficiency Syndrome(AIDS)—United States." *Morbidity and Mortality Weekly Report* 31 (Sept. 24): 507-14.

———. 1989a. *A Comprehensive Program to Prevent HIV Transmission, Fiscal Year 1989 Operating Plan.* Atlanta: Centers for Disease Control.

———. 1989b. *HIV/AIDS Surveillance Report* (Aug.). U.S. Department of Health and Human Services, Center for Infectious Diseases. Washington, D.C.: USGPO.

———. 1990a. *HIV/AIDS Surveillance Report* (Apr.). U.S. Department of Health and Human Services, Center for Infectious Diseases. Washington, D.C.: USGPO.

————. 1990b. "Update: Acquired Immunodeficiency Syndrome— United States, 1989." *Morbidity and Mortality Weekly Report* 39 (Feb. 9): 81-86.

Charles, K. 1985. "Factors in the Primary Prevention of AIDS in Gay and Bisexual Men." Doctoral Diss., California School of Professional Psychology, Berkeley.

Chiasson, M.A. et al. 1990 "Risk Factors for Human Immunodeficiency Virus Type I (HIV-1) Infection in Patients at a Sexually Transmitted Disease Clinic in New York City." *American Journal of Epidemiology* 131: 208-20.

Chiodi, F. et al. 1989. "Screening of African Sera Stored for More than 178 Years for HIV Antibodies by Site-Directed Serology." *European Journal of Epidemiology* 5, 1: 42-46.

Clavel, F., K. Mansinho, and S. Chamanet. 1987. "Human Immunodeficiency Virus Type 2 Infection Associated with AIDS in West Africa." *New England Journal of Medicine* 316: 1180-85.

Cliff, A. et al. 1981. *Spatial Diffusion: An Historical Geography of Epidemics in an Island Community.* Cambridge, England: Cambridge Univ. Press.

Clumeck, N. et al. 1984. "Acquired Immunodeficiency Syndrome in African Patients." *New England Journal of Medicine* 310: 492-97.

Coates, T.J., L. Temoshok, and J. Mandel. 1984. "Psychosocial Research Is Essential to Understanding and Treating AIDS." *American Psychologist* 39, 11: 1309-14.

———— et al. 1986. "AIDS: A Psychosocial Research Agenda." *Annals of Behavioral Medicine* 9, 2: 21-28.

———— et al. 1988. "AIDS Antibody Testing: Will It Stop the AIDS Epidemic? Will It Help People Infected with HIV?" *American Psychologist* 43: 859-64.

Coe, R.M. 1970. *Sociology of Medicine.* New York: McGraw-Hill.

Cohen, A.K. 1966. *Deviance and Control.* Englewood Cliffs, N.J.: Prentice-Hall.

Collins, P.H. 1986. "Learning from the Outsider Within: The Social Significance of Black Feminist Thought." *Social Problems* 33, 6 (Dec.): S14-S32.

Curran, J.W., and the Centers for Disease Control Task Force on Kaposi's Sarcoma and Opportunistic Infections. 1982. "Epidemiologic Aspects of the Current Outbreak of Kaposi's Sarcoma and Opportunistic Infections." *New England Journal of Medicine* 306 (Jan. 28): 248-52.

D'Aquila, R. et al. 1987. "HIV Seroprevalence among Connecticut

Intravenous Drug Users in 1986." Paper presented at the Third International Conference on AIDS. Washington, D.C., June 1-5.

Darrow, W.W. 1976. "Social and Behavioral Aspects of the Sexually Transmitted Diseases." In *Sexuality Today and Tomorrow: Contemporary Issues in Human Sexuality,* ed. S. Gordon and R.W. Libby, 134-54. North Scituate, Mass.: Duxbury.

———. 1977. "Social Stratification, Sexual Behavior, and the Sexually Transmitted Diseases." *Sexually Transmitted Diseases* 4: 228-36.

———. 1988. "Behavioral Changes in Response to AIDS." In *Symposium International de Reflexion sur le Sida,* 227-30. Paris: Berger-Levrault.

———, E.M. Gorman, and B.P. Glick. 1986. "The Social Origins of AIDS: Social Change, Sexual Behavior, and Disease Trends." In *The Social Dimensions of AIDS: Method and Theory,* ed. D.A. Feldman and T.M. Johnson, 95-107. New York: Praeger.

——— et al. 1989. "Human Immunodeficiency Virus Infection in Female Prostitutes." In *AIDS: 89-90: News and Views on Research and Control,* ed. G. de-The, 15-17. Paris: McGraw-Hill.

——— and the Centers for Disease Control Collaborative Group for the Study of HIV-1 in Selected Women. 1990. "Prostitution, Intravenous Drug Use, and HIV-1 in the United States." In *AIDS, Drugs and Prostitution,* ed. M.A. Plant, 18-40. London: Routledge.

DePerre, P. et al. 1984. "Acquired Immunodeficiency Syndrome in Rwanda." *Lancet* I: 62-69.

Des Jarlais, D., and S.R. Friedman. 1988. "The Psychology of Preventing AIDS among IV Drug Users: A Social Learning Conceptualization." *American Psychologist* (Nov.): 858-70.

——— et al. 1989. "HIV-1 Infection among Intravenous Drug Users in Manhattan, New York City, from 1977 through 1987." *Journal of the American Medical Association* 261, 7: 108-12.

Desmyter, J. et al. 1986. "Origin of AIDS." *British Medical Journal* 293: 1306.

Dhooper, S., and D. Royse. 1989. "Rural Attitudes about AIDS: A Statewide Survey." *Human Services in the Rural Environment* 13, 1 (Summer): 17-22.

DiClemente, R., J. Zorn, and L. Temoskok. 1986. "Adolescents and AIDS: A Survey of Knowledge, Attitudes and Beliefs about AIDS in San Francisco." *American Journal of Public Health* 76: 1443-45.

Drotman, D.P., and J.W. Curran. 1984. "AIDS: An Epidemiologic Overview." In *AIDS: The Epidemic of Kaposi's Sarcoma and Opportunistic Infections,* ed. A.E. Friedman-Kien and L.J. Laubenstein, 279-86. New York: Masson.

Drucker, E. 1986. Unpublished data analysis based on New York State Hospital Reporting System.

—— et al. 1987. "Hospital Utilization Patterns and Changes for the Case of Inner-City AIDS Patients: By Risk Group, Sex, and Race/Ethnicity." Paper presented at the Third International Conference on AIDS. Washington, D.C.: June 1-5.

—— et al. 1988. "IV Drug Users with AIDS in New York City: A Study of Dependent Children, Housing, and Drug Addiction Treatment." Unpublished paper. New York: Albert Einstein College of Medicine, Department of Epidemiology and Social Medicine.

—— and S.H. Vermund. 1989. "Estimating Population Prevalence of Human Immunodeficiency Virus Infection in Urban Areas with High Rates of Intravenous Drug Use: A Model of the Bronx in 1988." *American Journal of Epidemiology*, 130, 1 (July): 133-42.

—— et al. 1989a. "Heterosexual Contact of 429 Pregnant Non-IV Drug Using Women in the South Bronx, New York, in 1988." Paper presented at the Fifth International Conference on AIDS. Montreal, Canada, June 4-9.

—— et al. 1989b. "Increasing Rate of Pneumonia Hospitalizations in the Bronx: A Sentinel Indicator for Human Immunodeficiency Virus." *International Journal of Epidemiology* 18, 4: 926-33.

—— 1990. "Epidemic in the War Zone: AIDS and Community Survival in New York City." *International Journal of Health Services* 20(4): 601-15.

Duesberg, P. 1987. "Retroviruses as Carcinogens and Pathogens: Expectations and Reality." *Cancer Research* 47: 1199-1220.

Edwards, D. 1987. "Heterosexuals and AIDS: Mixed Messages." *Science News* 132 (July): 60-61.

Eisenhandler, J. 1989. "The HIV Experience of Empire Blue Cross and Blue Shield." Unpublished paper.

—— and E. Drucker. 1990. "Estimating the Prevalence of IV Drug Use and HIV Infection among Subscribers of a Large Private Health Insurance Plan in the New York Area." Abstract presented at the Sixth International Conference on AIDS. San Francisco.

Ellrodt, A. et al. 1984. "Isolation of Human T-Lymphotroic Retrovirus (LAV) from Azairian Married Couple, One with AIDS, One with Prodomes." *Lancet* II: 1383-85.

Ernst, J. 1990. Personal communication, with E. Drucker, based on unpublished data from the Bronx Lebanon Hospital Center, New York.

Essex, M. 1989. "Origins of AIDS." In *AIDS Etiology, Diagnosis, Treatment and Prevention,* ed. V.T. DeVita, Jr., S. Hellman, and S. Rosenberg, 3-10. Philadelphia: Lippincott.

———— and P. Kanki. 1988. "The Origins of the AIDS Virus." *Scientific American* 259: 64-71.

Executive Intelligence Review. 1988. "The U.S.S.R. and the Origin of the AIDS Virus." *AIDS: Global Showdown: Mankind's Total Victory or Total Defeat.* Part VII, 119-26. Washington D.C.

Farmer, P. 1990. "AIDS and Accusation: Haiti, Haitians, and the Geography of Blame." In *Culture and AIDS,* ed. D.A. Feldman. New York: Praeger.

Farthing, C., S. Brown, and R. Staughton. 1988. *Color Atlas of AIDS and HIV Diseases.* 2d. ed. Chicago: Year Book Medical Publishers, Inc.

Fee, E. 1988. "Sin vs. Science: Venereal Disease in Twentieth Century Baltimore." In *AIDS: The Burdens of History,* ed. E. Fee and D. Fox. Berkeley: Univ. of California Press.

Feldman, D.A. 1990a. "Assessing Viral, Parasitic and Sociocultural Cofactors Affecting HIV-1 Transmission in Rwanda." In *Culture and AIDS,* ed. D.A. Feldman. New York: Praeger.

————. 1990b. "Introduction: Culture and AIDS." In *Culture and AIDS,* ed. D.A. Feldman. New York: Praeger.

Flahault, A., and A.J. Valleron. 1989. "The Role of Air Transport in the Global Spread of HIV Infection." Manuscript 15.

Flora, J., and C. Thorenson. 1988. "Reducing the Risk of AIDS in Adolescents." *American Psychologist* 43: 965-70.

Foster, S., and W. Gorr. 1985. "Forecasting the Geographic Distribution of Primary Care Physicians: An Application of Spatial Adaptive Filtering." *Proceedings of the Sixteenth Annual Pittsburgh Conference on Modeling and Simulation* (Apr.): 87-91.

———— and ————. 1986. "An Adaptive Filter for Estimating Spatially Varying Parameters: An Application to Modeling Policy Hours Spent in Response to Calls for Service." *Management Science* 32: 878-89.

Friedson, E. 1976. *Doctoring Together: A Study of Professional Social Control.* New York: Elsevier.

Friedman, S.R. et al. 1987. "AIDS and Self-Organization Among Intravenous Drug Users." *International Journal of the Addictions* 22, 3: 201-19.

———— et al. 1988. "Racial Aspects of the AIDS Epidemic." *California Sociologist* 11, 1-2 (Winter/Summer): 55-68.

Froland, S. et al. 1988. "HIV-1 Infection in a Norwegian Family Before 1970." *Lancet* II: 1344-45.

Gagnon, J.H. and W. Simon. 1973. *Sexual Conduct: The Social Sources of Human Sexuality.* Chicago: Aldine.

Gail, M., and R. Brookmeyer. 1988. "Methods for Projecting Course of Acquired Immunodeficiency Syndrome Epidemic." *Journal of the National Cancer Institute* 80: 900-911.

Gallo, R.C., and L. Montagnier. 1989. "The AIDS Epidemic." In *The Science of AIDS,* ed. J. Piel, 1-11. New York: W.H. Freeman.

Gardner, L. et al. 1989. "Spatial Diffusion of the Human Immunodeficiency Virus Infection Epidemic in the United States, 1985-87." *Annals of the Association of American Geographers* 79, 1, (Mar.): 25-43.

Garry, R. et al. 1988. "Documentation of an AIDS Virus Infection in the United States in 1968." *Journal of the American Medical Association* 260: 2085-87.

Gonzalez, J. et al. 1987. "True HIV-1 Infection in a Pygmy." *Lancet* I: 1490.

Good, C. 1988. "Traditional Healers and AIDS Management." In *AIDS in Africa: The Social and Policy Impact,* ed. N. Miller and R.C. Rockwell, 97-114. Lewiston, N.Y.: Edwin Mellon.

Gorr, W., and C. Hsu. 1985. "An Adaptive Filtering Procedure for Estimating Regression Quantiles." *Management Science* 31: 1019-29.

Gould, P.R. 1969. *Spatial Diffusion.* Washington, D.C.: Association of American Geographers.

————. 1989. "Geographic Dimensions of the AIDS Epidemic." *Professional Geographer* 41, 1 (Feb.): 71-78.

————, W. Gorr, and E. Casetti, 1988. *Understanding and Predicting the AIDS Epidemic in Geographic Space.* University Park, Pa.: The Penn State-Carnegie Mellon-Ohio State Consortium.

————, D. DiBiase, and J. Kabel. 1989. *The Diffusion of AIDS.* Twenty-minute video-tape made in conjunction with WPSX-TV. University Park, Pa.

Gould, R.E. 1988. "Reassuring News about AIDS: A Doctor Tells Why You May Not Be at Risk." *Cosmopolitan,* Jan., 146, 147, 204.

Greaves, W.L. 1987. "The Black Community." In *AIDS and the Law,* ed. H.L. Dalton, 281-89. New Haven, Conn.: Yale Univ. Press.

Greifinger, R. 1990. "New York State Department of Corrections Data." Presented at the Fourth Montefiore Symposium on AIDS. New York City, Jan. 23.

Grossman, M. 1988. "Children with AIDS." In *AIDS: Principles, Practices and Politics,* ed. I. Corless and M. Pittman-Lindeman. Washington, D.C.: Hemisphere.

Hammonds, E. 1987. "Race, Sex, AIDS: The Construction of 'Other.'" *Radical America* 20, 6.

Hamid, A. 1990. "The Political Economy of Crack-Related Violence." *Contemporary Drug Problems* 17: 31-78.

Haq, C. 1988. "Data on AIDS in Africa: An Assessment." In *AIDS in Africa: The Social and Policy Impact,* ed. N. Miller and R.C. Rockwell, 9-30. Lewiston, N.Y.: Edwin Mellon.

Hayes, J., Jr., R. Marlink, and S. Hardawi. 1989. "HIV-/Related Disease in Africa." In *Pathology and Pathophysiology of AIDS and HIV-Related Diseases,* ed. S. Harawi and C. O'Hara, 443-58. St. Louis: Mosby.

Heagarty, M.C. 1987. "AIDS: A View from the Trenches." *Issues in Science and Technology* (Winter): 111-17.

Health Systems Agency. 1989. *New York City AIDS Task Force Report.* New York: New York City Department of Health.

Herskovits, M.J. 1971 [1937]. *Life in a Haitian Valley.* New York: Knopf.

Hessol, N.A. et al. 1988. "Seroconversion to HIV among Homosexual and Bisexual Men Who Participated in Hepatitis B Vaccine Trials." Paper presented at the Fourth International Conference on AIDS, Stockholm, Sweden, June.

—— et al. 1989. "Prevalence, Incidence and Progression of Human Immunodeficiency Virus Infection in Homosexual and Bisexual Men in Hepatitis B. Vaccine Trials." *American Journal of Epidemiology* 130, 6: 1167-75.

Hira, S. 1989. "Perinatal Transmission." Paper presented at the Second National STD/AIDS Seminar. Lusaka, Zambia, Mar.

Horrigan, A. 1988. "AIDS and the Catholic Church." In *The Social Impact of AIDS in the U. S.,* ed. R.A. Berk. Cambridge, Mass. Abt.

Horsburgh, D.C., Jr., and S. Homberg. 1988. "The Global Distribution of Human Immunodeficiency Virus Type 2 (HIV-2) Infection." *Transfusion* 28, 2: 192-95.

Hoyle, F., and N.C. Wickramasingke. 1990. "Sunspots and Influenza." *Nature* 343: 304.

Intergovernmental AIDS Reports. 1989. *National Survey of State Funding for AIDS* 2 (3A):1-12.

Jaffe, H.W. et al. 1983. "National Case-Control Study of Kaposi's Sarcoma and Pneumoncystis carinii Pneumonia in Homosexual Men: Part 1, Epidemiologic Results." *Annals of Internal Medicine* 99 (Aug.: 145-51.

Johnson, P., D. Munoz, and J. Pares. 1988. "Multicultural Concerns and AIDS Action: Creating an Alternative." *Radical America* 21, 2-3: 24-33.

Joint Task Force of the National Association of Community Health Centers and the National Rural Health Association. 1989. "Health Care in Rural America: The Crisis Unfolds." *Journal of Public Health Policy* 10, 1 (Spring): 99-116.

Joseph, J. et al. 1987. "Behavioral Risk Reduction in a Cohort of

Homosexual Men: Two Year Follow-up." Paper presented at the Third International Conference on AIDS, Washington, D.C.

Kangas, L.W., J.R. Harris, and J.D. Shelton. 1989. "The Supply of, and Demand for, Condoms to Prevent HIV Transmission in Developing Countries." Poster session presented at the Fifth International Conference on AIDS, Montreal, Canada, June.

Kanki, P.J., J. Alroy, and M. Essex. 1985. "Isolation of T-Lymphotropic Retrovirus Related to HTLV-III/LAV from Wild Caught African Green Monkeys." *Science* 230: 951-54.

———— et al. 1986. "New Human T-lymphotrophic Retrovirus Related to Simian T-lymphotropic Virus Type III (STLV-III AGM)." *Science* 238-43, (Apr. 11).

Kantner, H., and G. Pankey. 1987. "Evidence for a Euro-American Origin of Human Immunodeficiency Virus (HIV)." *Journal of the National Medical Association* 79, 10: 1068-72.

Kaplan, Helen S. 1987. *The Real Truth about Women with AIDS: How to Eliminate Risks Without Giving Up Love and Sex.* New York: Simon and Schuster.

Kaplan, Howard, ed. 1983. *Psychosocial Stress: Trends in Theory and Research.* New York: Academic.

Kashamura, A. 1973. *Famille, Sexualité et Culture: Essai sur les Moneurs Sexuelles et les Cultures des Peuples des Grands Lacs Africains.* Paris: Payot.

Kaslow, R.A. et al. 1989. "No Evidence for a Role of Alcohol or Other Psychoactive Drugs in Accelerating Immunodeficiency in HIV-1 Positive Individuals." *Journal of American Medical Association* 261, 23: 3424-29.

Keeling, R. 1989. "HIV in American University Populations." Presentation at the Ritenour Health Center, Pennsylvania State University, University Park, Mar.

Kirp, D., and Associates. 1989. *Learning by Heart: AIDS and Schoolchildren in America's Communities.* New Brunswick, N.J.: Rutgers Univ. Press.

Kitchen, L.W. 1987. "AIDS in Africa: Knowns and Unknowns." *CSIS Africa Notes* 74: 1-4.

Klovdahl, A.S. 1985. "Social Networks and the Spread of Infectious Diseases: The AIDS Example." *Social Science and Medicine* 21, 11: 1203-16.

Koch, P., and S. Peckman. 1989. *An Assessment of Knowledge, Attitudes and Beliefs among Eleventh Grade Public School Students.* University Park, Pa.: College of Health Education.

Konotey-Ahulu, F. 1987. "AIDS in Africa: Misinformation and Disinformation." *Lancet* II: 206-7.

Lambert, B. 1989a. "In Spite of Crisis, New York Lacks Basic Services for AIDS Patients." *New York Times* (Jan. 3).

———. 1989b. "Aids Legacy: A Growing Generation of Orphans." *New York Times* (July 17): A1 +.

———. 1989c. "Hospital Policy Is Said to Hurt AIDS Patients." *New York Times* (Sept. 8): B2.

———. 1989d. "AIDS Battler Gives Needles Illicitly to Addicts." *New York Times* (Nov. 20): A1.

———. 1990. AIDS Travels Air-Bridge to Puerto Rico. *New York Times* (June 15): A8, G1.

Laws, J., and P. Schwartz. 1977. *Sexual Scripts: The Social Construction of Female Sexuality.* Hinsdale, Ill. Dryden.

Lee, F. 1989. "Black Doctors Urge Study of Factors in Risk of AIDS." *New York Times* (July 21): B7.

Leibowitch, J. 1985. *A Strange Virus of Unknown Origin,* translated from French by R. Howard. New York: Ballatine.

Leishman, K. 1987. "Heterosexuals and AIDS." *Atlantic Monthly,* Feb.

Lemp, G.F. et al. 1988. "Projections of AIDS Morbidity and Mortality in San Francisco Using Epidemic Models." Paper presented at the Fourth International Conference on AIDS, Stockholm, Sweden, June.

Leonidas, J., and N. Hyppolite. 1983. "Haiti and the Acquired Immunodeficiency Syndrome." *Annals of Internal Medicine* 98: 1021.

Lepage, P. et al. 1986. "Are Medical Infections a Risk Factor for HIV Infection in Children?" *Lancet* II: 1103-4.

Lexington Herald-Leader. Lexington, Kentucky.

Li, Y. et al. 1989. "Extensive Genetic Variability of Simiao Immunodeficiency Virus from African Green Monkeys." *Journal of Virology* 63: 1800-1802.

Lifson, A., R. Stall, and W. Winkelstein. 1989. "Continued Seroconversion for HIV Antibody Among Homosexual and Bisexual Men." *San Francisco Epidemiologic Bulletin* 5, 8: 35-37.

Longini, I.M., Jr. et al. 1989. "Statistical Analysis of the Stages of HIV Infection Using a Markov Model." *Statistics in Medicine* 8, 7 (July): 831-43.

———, P. Fine, and S. Thacker. 1986. "Predicting the Global Spread of New Infectious Agents." *American Journal of Epidemiology* 123: 383-91.

Louisville Courier-Journal. Louisville, Kentucky.

Lwegaba, A. 1988. Personal communication with D.A. Feldman.

Lyons, S., B. Schoub, and G. McGillivray. 1985. "Lack of Evidence of

HTLV-III in Southern Africa." *New England Journal of Medicine* 314: 1257-58.

McClure, M., and T. Schulz. 1989. "Origin of HIV." *British Medical Journal* (May 13).

MacFarlane, M.A. 1989. "Equal Opportunities—Protecting the Rights of AIDS Linked Children in the Classroom." *American Journal of Law and Medicine* 14, 4: 377-430.

McKusick, L. et al. 1985. "Reported Changes in the Sexual Behavior of Men at Risk for AIDS, San Francisco, 1982-1984: The AIDS Behavioral Research Project." *Public Health Reports* 100: 622-29.

MacMahon, B., and T.F. Pugh. 1970. *Epidemiology: Principles and Methods.* Boston: Little, Brown.

Makridakis, J., and S. Wheelwright. 1977. "Adaptive Filtering: An Integrated Autoregressive-Moving Average Filter for Time Series Forecasting." *Operations Research Quarterly* 28: 425-37.

Mann, J.M. 1987. "The Epidemiology of LAV/HTLV-III in Africa." In *Acquired Immunodeficiency Syndrome,* ed. J. Gluckman and E. Vilmer, 131-36. Amsterdam: Elsevier.

———. 1988. "The Global Picture of AIDS." *Journal of Acquired Immune Deficiency Syndromes* 1: 209-16.

——— et al. 1986. "Risk Factors for HIV Seropositivity Among Children 1-24 Months Old in Kinshasa, Zaire." *Lancet* II: 654-56.

Mason, B. 1989. Personal communication with Edwin Hackney.

Masters, W.H., V.E. Johnson, and R.C. Kolodny. 1988. *Crisis: Heterosexual Behavior in the Age of AIDS.* New York: Grove.

Mays, V.M., and S.D. Cochran. 1988. "Issues in the Perception of AIDS Risk and Risk Reduction Activities by Black and Hispanic/Latina Women." *American Psychologist* 43, 11 (Nov.): 949-57.

Menendez, B.S. et al. 1990. "AIDS Mortality Among Puerto Ricans and Other Hispanics in New York City, 1981-1987." *Journal of Acquired Immune Deficiency Syndromes* 3: 644-48.

Merritt, G. 1988. "U.S. Agency for International Development's HIV/AIDS Prevention Programs in Africa." Paper presented at the annual meeting of the American Association for the Advancement of Sciences, Boston, Mass. Feb.

———, W. Lyerly, and J. Thomas. 1988. "The HIV/AIDS Pandemic in Africa: Issues of Donor Strategy." In *AIDS in Africa: The Social and Policy Impact,* ed. N. Miller and R.C. Rockwell, 115-30. Lewiston, N.Y.: Edwin Mellon.

Merton, R.K. 1965. "Notes on Problem-Finding in Sociology." In *Sociology Today: Problems and Prospects,* ed. R.K. Merton, L. Broom, and L.S. Cottrell, Jr., ix-xxxiv. New York: Harper Torchbooks.

Metraux, A. 1972. *Voodoo in Haiti*. Trans. H. Chateris. New York: Schocken.

Moeller, R., and G. Bachman. 1988. "Assessment of Adolescents at Risk for HIV Infection." *Medical Aspects of Human Sexuality:* 20-32.

Moore, A., and R. LeBaron. 1986. "The Case for a Haitian Origin of AIDS Epidemic." In *The Social Dimensions of AIDS: Method and Theory,* ed. D.A. Feldman and R. Johnson, 77-93. New York: Praeger.

Moore, J., and M. Devitt. 1989. "The Paradox of Deviance in Addicted Mexican American Mothers." *Gender & Society* 3, 1 (Mar.): 53-70.

Morrill, R. 1968. "Waves of Spatial Diffusion." *Journal of Regional Science* 8: 1-18.

Moulton, J.M. et al. 1987. "Attributes of Blame and Responsibility in Relation to Distress and Health Behavior Change in People with AIDS and AIDS-Related Complex." *Journal of Applied Social Psychology* 17: 493-506.

Mulder, C. 1988. "Human AIDS Virus not from Monkeys." *Nature* 333: 396.

Murphy, A. 1988. "Women with AIDS: Sexual Ethics in an Epidemic." In *AIDS: Principles, Practices, and Politics,* ed. I. Corless and M. Pittman-Lindeman. Washington, D.C.: Hemisphere.

Nahmias, A. et al. 1986. "Evidence for Human Infection with an HTLV III/LAV-like Virus in Central Africa." *Lancet* I: 1279-80.

Najera, R., M. Herrera, and R. Andres. 1987. "Human Immunodeficiency Virus and Related Retroviruses." *Western Journal of Medicine* 147i, 6: 702-8.

National Academy of Sciences. Institute of Medicine. 1986a. *Confronting AIDS: Directions for Public Health, Health Care, and Research*. Washington, D.C.: National Academy.

————. 1986b. *Mobilizing Against AIDS*. Cambridge, Mass.: Harvard Univ. Press.

————. Committee on AIDS Research and the Behavioral, Social and Statistical Sciences, National Research Council. 1989. *AIDS Sexual Behavior and Intravenous Drug Abuse*. Washington, D.C.: National Academy.

National Association of State Boards of Education. 1989. "Someone At School Has AIDS." Washington, D.C.

National Center of Health Statistics. 1982. "Monthly Vital Statistics Report." *Advance Report of Final Natality, 1980* 31, 8.

New York City Department of Health. 1990. *AIDS Surveillance Update,* Feb. 28.

New York City Department of Health AIDS Surveillance. 1986.

"The AIDS Epidemic in New York City, 1981-1984." *American Journal of Epidemiology* 123: 1013-25.

New York Times. 1989. "Pregnant Women to Get AIDS Drug in Test." July 11: C2.

Ngugi, E.N. et al. 1988. "Prevention of Transmission of Human Immunodeficiency Virus in Africa: Effectiveness of Condom Promotion and Health Education Among Prostitutes." *Lancet* II: 887-90.

Norwood, C. 1987. *Advice for Life: A Woman's Guide to AIDS Risks and Prevention.* New York: Pantheon.

Novick, L.F. et al. 1989. "HIV Seroprevalence in Newborns in New York State." *Journal of the American Medical Association* 261: 1745-50.

Nzilambi, N. et al. 1988. "The Prevalence of Infection With Human Immunodeficiency Virus Over a Ten-Year Period in Rural Zaire." *New England Journal of Medicine* 318, 5 (Feb. 4): 276-79.

Okware, S. 1987. "Towards a National AIDS-Control Program in Uganda." *Western Journal of Medicine* 147, 6: 276.

O'Connell, M. 1980. "Comparative Estimates of Teenage Illegitimacy in the United States, 1940-44 to 1970-74." *Demography* 17 (Feb.): 13-24.

Openshaw, S. et al. 1989. "Empirical Study of Confidentiality Risks in the Release of Mircocensus Data," Manuscript: 10. Newcastle upon Tyne, England: Center for Urban and Regional Development Studies.

O'Reilly, K.R. et al. 1989. "Perceived Community Norms and Risk Reduction: Behavior Change in a Cohort of Gay Men." Paper presented at the Fifth International Conference on AIDS, Montreal, Canada, June.

Pape, J., and W. Johnson. 1989. "HIV-1 Infection and AIDS in Haiti." In *Epidemiology of AIDS*, ed. R. Kaslow and D. Francis, 221-30. New York: Oxford Univ. Press.

Patton, C. 1985. *Sex, Germs and AIDS.* Boston: South End.

Piot, P. et al. 1984. "Acquired Immunodeficiency Syndrome in a Heterosexual Population in Zaire." *Lancet* II: 65-69.

Piot, R., and R. Colebunders. 1987. "Clinical Manifestations and the Natural History of HIV Infection in Adults." *Western Journal of Medicine* 147: 709-12.

Presidential Commission on the Human Immunodeficiency Virus Epidemic. 1988. *Report of the Presidential Commission on the Human Immunodeficiency Virus Epidemic.* Washington, D.C.: USGPO.

Quinn, T., and J. Mann. 1989. "HIV-1 Infection and AIDS in Africa." In *The Epidemiology of AIDS*, ed. R. Kaslow and D. Francis, 194-219. New York: Oxford Univ. Press.

Richardson, D. 1988. *Women and AIDS.* New York: Methuen.

Robins, L. 1980. "The Natural History of Drug Abuse." In *Theories of Drug Abuse.* ed. D. Lettieri, M. Sayers, and H. Wallerstein Pearson, 215-224. Washington, D.C.: USGPO.

Rosenbaum, M. 1981. *Women on Heroin.* New Brunswick, N.J.: Rutgers Univ. Press.

Rothman, B.K. 1987. "Reproduction." In *Analyzing Gender,* ed. B. Hess and M.M. Ferree. Newbury Park, Calif.: Sage.

Rounds, K. 1988. "AIDS in Rural Areas: Challenges to Providing Care." *Social Work* (May-June): 257-61.

Royse, D. et al. 1987. "Undergraduate and Graduate Students' Attitudes Towards AIDS." *Psychology Reports* 60: 1185-86.

Rvachev, L., and I. Longini. 1985. "A Mathematical Model for the Global Spread of Influenza." *Mathematical Biosciences* 75: 3-22.

Ryder, R.W. et al. 1989. "Perinatal Transmission of the Human Immunodeficiency Virus Type 1 to Infants of Seropositive Women in Zaire." *New England Journal of Medicine* 320 (June 22): 1637-42.

Sabatier, R. 1987. "Social, Cultural and Demographic Aspects of AIDS." *Western Journal of Medicine* 147, 6: 713-15.

Schmidt, N. 1988. "Resources on the Social Impact of AIDS in Africa." In *AIDS in Africa,* ed. N. Miller and R. Rockwell, 239-43. Lewiston, N.Y.: Edwin Mellon.

Schneider, B.E. 1988. "Gender, Sexuality and AIDS: Social Responses and Consequences." In *the Social Impact of AIDS in the U.S.,* ed. R.A. Berk, Cambridge, Mass.: Abt.

———. 1989. "AIDS and Class, Gender and Race Relations." Paper presented at the annual meeting of the American Sociological Association, San Francisco, August 1989.

——— and M. Gould. 1987. "Female Sexuality: Looking Back Into the Future." In *Analyzing Gender,* ed. B. Hess and M.M. Ferree. Newbury Park, Calif.: Sage.

Schreeder, M.T. et al. 1982. "Hepatitis B in Homosexual Men: Prevalence of Infection and Factors Related to Transmission." *Journal of Infectious Diseases* 146 (July): 7-15.

Scott, J. 1989. "Family Clinic Funding Cutbacks Hit Poor Hardest, Officials Say." *Los Angeles Times* (July 28): 3.

Selik, R.M., K.B. Castro, and M. Pappaioanou. 1988. "Racial/Ethnic Differences in the Risk of AIDS in the United States." *American Journal of Public Health* 78, 12 (Dec.: 1539-45.

——— et al. 1989. "Birthplace and the Risk of AIDS Among Hispanics in the United States." *American Journal of Public Health* 79: 836-39.

Selwyn, P.A. et al. 1989. "Knowledge of HIV Antibody Status and Decisions to Continue or Terminate Pregnancy Among Intravenous

Drug Users." *Journal of the American Medical Association* 261, 24 (June 23-30): 3567-71.

Shafer, M. 1988. "High Risk Behavior During Adolescence." In *AIDS in Children, Adolescents and Heterosexual Adults,* ed. R. Schinazi and A. Nahmais, 329-34. New York: Elsevier.

Shannon, G.S., and G.F. Pyle. 1989. "The Origin and Diffusion of AIDS: A View from Medical Geography." *Annals of the Association of American Geographers* 79, 1 (Mar.): 1-24.

——, G.F. Pyle, and R. Bashur. 1990. *The Geography of AIDS.* New York: Guilford.

Shaw, N.S. 1988. "Preventing AIDS among Women: The Role of Community Organizing." *Socialist Review* 18, 4 (Oct.-Dec.).

—— and L. Paleo. 1986. "Women and AIDS." In *What to do about AIDS: Physicians and Mental Health Professionals Discuss the Issues,* ed. L. McKusick. Berkeley: Univ. of California Press.

Shilts, R. 1988. *And the Band Played On: Politics, People and the AIDS Epidemic.* New York: Penguin.

Sisk, J., M. Hewitt, and K. Metcalf. 1988. "The Effectiveness of AIDS Education." *Health Affairs:* 37-51.

Smith, H. 1983. "AIDS: The Haitian Connection." *MD:* 46-52.

Sonenstein, F.L., J.H. Pleck, and L.C. Ku. 1989. "Sexual Activity, Condom Use and AIDS Awareness among Adolescent Males." *Family Planning Perspectives* 21 (July): 152-58.

Spitzer, P. and N. Weiver. 1989. "Transmission of HIV Infection from a Woman to a Man by Oral Sex." *New England Journal of Medicine* 320: 251.

Stall, R., T. Coates, and C. Hoff. 1988. "Behavioral Risk Reduction for HIV Infection among Gay and Bisexual Men: A Review of Results from the United States." *American Psychologist* 43, 11: 878-85.

—— et al. 1986. "Alcohol and Drug Use During Sexual Activity and Compliance with Safe Sex Guidelines for AIDS: The AIDS Behavioral Research Project." *Health Education Quarterly* 13: 359-71.

—— and D. Ostrow. 1989. "Intravenous Drug Use, the Combination of Drugs and Sexual Activity and HIV Infection among Gay and Bisexual Men: The San Francisco Men's Health Study." *Journal of Drug Issues* 19, 1: 57-73.

—— and J. Paul. 1989. "Changes in Sexual Risk for Infection with the Human Immunodeficiency Virus among Gay and Bisexual Men in San Francisco." Report to the Global Programme on AIDS in support of the Consultation on Risk Reduction among Gay and Bisexual Men. Geneva, Switzerland, May.

Steigbigel, N. et al. 1987. "Heterosexual Transmission of Infection and Disease by the Human Immunodeficiency Virus (HIV)." Paper presented at the Third International Conference on AIDS. Washington, D.C., June 1-5.

Stoneburner, R.L. et al. 1988. "A Larger Spectrum of Severe HIV-1 Related Disease in Intravenous Drug Users in New York City." *Science* 242, 4880: 916-19.

Strunin, L., and R. Hingson. 1987. "Acquired Immunodeficiency Syndrome and Adolescents: Knowledge, Beliefs, Attitudes and Behavior." *Pediatrics* 79: 825-28.

Taravella, S. 1989. "Women with AIDS Find Abortions Hard to Get in New York. *"Modern Health Care* 19, 33 (Aug. 18).

Terry, J. 1989. "The Body Invaded: Medical Surveillance of Women as Reproducers." *Socialist Review* 3: 13-43.

Thompson, K. 1980. "A Comparison of Black and White Adolescents' Beliefs about Having Children." *Journal of Marriage and the Family* 42 (Feb.): 133-40.

Torrey, B.B., P.O. Way, and P.M. Rowe. 1988. "Epidemiology of HIV and AIDS in Africa: Emerging Issues and Social Implications." In *AIDS in Africa: The Social and Policy Impact,* ed. N. Miller and R.C. Rockwell, 31-54. Lewiston, N.Y.: Edwin Mellon.

Tumani, C. et al. 1989. "Clinical Characterization of HIV-2 Disease in West Africa." Poster session presented at the Fifth International Conference on AIDS. Montreal, Canada, June.

U.S. Congress. 1990a. House Report to accompany H.R. 2990. Departments of Labor, Health and Human Services, and Education and Related Agencies Appropriation Bill.

———. 1990b. Senate Report 101-127 to accompany H.R. 2990. Departments of Labor, Health and Human Services, and Education and Related Agencies Appropriation Bill.

Van de Perre, P. et al. 1984. "Acquired Immunodeficiency Syndrome in Rwanda." *Lancet* II: 62-65.

Vermund, S.H. et al. 1989. "Acquired Immunodeficiency Syndrome Among Adolescents." *American Journal of Diseases of Children* 143: 1220-25.

Vladeck, B. 1990. "Worst-Case Scenarios." *President's Letter,* United Hospital Fund, Feb.

Volberding, P.A. et al. 1990. "Zidovudine in Asymptomatic Human Immunodeficiency Virus Infection." *New England Journal of Medicine* 322: 941-49.

Von Reyn, C. and J. Mann. 1987. "Global Epidemiology." *Western Journal of Medicine* 147, 6: 694-701.

Waite, G. 1988. "The Politics of Disease: The AIDS Virus and Africa." In *AIDS in Africa,* ed. N. Miller and R. Rockwell, 145-64. Lewiston, N.Y.: Edwin Mellon.

Waldrop, M.W. 1989. "NIDA Aims to Fight Drugs With Drugs." *Science* 245, 4925: 1443-44.

Wawer, M. 1988. Personal communication with D.A. Feldman.

Webster, P. 1984. "The Forbidden: Eroticism and Taboo." In *Pleasure and Danger,* ed. C. Vance. Boston: Routledge and Kegan Paul.

Williams, T.M. 1989. *The Cocaine Kids: The Inside Story of a Teenage Drug Ring.* Reading, Mass.: Addison-Wesley.

Winkelstein, W. et al. 1987. "The San Francisco Men's Health Study: III. Reduction in Human Immunodeficiency Virus Transmission among Homosexual/Bisexual Men, 1982-86." *American Journal of Public Health* 77, 6: 685-89.

Winkenwerder, W.A., A.R. Kessler, and R.M. Stolec. 1989. "Federal Spending for Illness Caused by the Human Immunodeficiency Virus." *New England Journal of Medicine* 320, 24: 1598-1603.

Winslow, C.E.A. 1980. *The Conquest of Epidemic Disease.* Madison: Univ. of Wisconsin Press.

Worth, D., and R. Rodriguez. 1987. "Latina Women and AIDS." *Radical America* 20, 6 (Nov.).

Yeager, R. 1988. "Historical and Ecological Ramifications for AIDS in Eastern and Central Africa." In *AIDS in Africa,* ed. N. Miller and R. Rockwell, 71-81. Lewiston, N.Y.: Edwin Mellon.

Young, E., P. Koch, and D. Preston. 1989. "AIDS and Homosexuality: A Longitudinal Study of Knowledge and Attitude Change Among Rural Nurses." *Public Health Nursing* 6: 189-96.

Zelnik, M., and J.F. Kantner. 1980. "Sexual Activity, Contraceptive Use and Pregnancy among Metropolitan-Area Teenagers: 1971-1979." *Family Planning Perspectives* 12 (Sept.-Oct.): 230-37.

Zimmerman, M.K. 1987. "The Women's Health Movement: A Critique of Medical Enterprise and the Position of Women." In *Analyzing Gender,* ed. B. Hess and M. Marx, 442-72. Newbury Park, Calif.: Sage.

Zuckerman, A. 1986. "AIDS and Insects." *British Medical Journal* 292: 1094-95.

Contributors

William W. Darrow, Ph.D., is chief of the Social and Behavioral Studies Section, Epidemiology Branch, Division of HIV/AIDS, Center for Infectious Diseases, Centers for Disease Control, Public Health Service, U.S. Department of Health and Human Services, Atlanta, Georgia.

Ernest Drucker, Ph.D., is director of the Division of Community Health and professor, Department of Epidemiology and Social Medicine, Montefiore Medical Center, Albert Einstein College of Medicine, Bronx, New York.

Douglas A. Feldman, Ph.D., is associate professor in the Department of Epidemiology and Public Health, University of Miami Medical Center, Miami, Florida.

Peter Gould, Ph.D., is Evan Pugh Professor of Geography, Department of Geography, Pennsylvania State University, University Park.

Edwin Hackney, M.S.W., is coordinator of Out-patient Substance Abuse Services, Bluegrass East Comprehensive Care Center, Lexington, Kentucky.

Beth E. Schneider, Ph.D., is associate professor in the Department of Sociology, University of California, Santa Barbara.

Gary W. Shannon, Ph.D., is professor in the Department of Geography, University of Kentucky, Lexington.

William F. Skinner, Ph.D., is associate professor in the Department of Sociology, University of Kentucky, Lexington.

Ronald Stall, Ph.D., M.P.H., is an assistant adjunct professor at the Department of Epidemiology and Biostatistics and works at the Center for AIDS Prevention Studies, University of California, San Francisco.

Richard Ulack, Ph.D., is professor and chair of the Department of Geography, University of Kentucky, Lexington.

Ernestine Vanderveen, Ph.D., is associate director, Division of Basic Research, National Institute on Alcohol Abuse and Alcoholism, Department of Health and Human Services, Rockville, Maryland.